Men's Fitness
magazine

Workout Manual

Editor Jon Lipsey
Design Ian Jackson
Subeditor Chris Miller

 © Copyright Dennis Publishing
Ltd. Licensed by Felden 2011 MAG**BOOK**

Managing Director **James Burnay**
Digital Production Manager **Nicky Baker**
Bookazine Manager **Dharmesh Mistry**
Operations Director **Robin Ryan**
Managing Director of Advertising
Julian Lloyd-Evans
Newstrade Director **David Barker**
Chief Operating Officer **Brett Reynolds**
Group Finance Director **Ian Leggett**
Chief Executive Officer **James Tye**
Chairman **Felix Dennis**

The 'MagBook' brand is a trademark of Dennis Publishing Ltd.
30 Cleveland St, London W1T 4JD. Company registered in England.
All material © Dennis Publishing Ltd, licensed by Felden 2011,
and may not be reproduced in whole or part without the
consent of the publishers.

Workout Manual ISBN 1-78106-003-7
To license this product please contact Hannah Heagney on
+44 (0) 20 7907 6134 or email hannah_heagney@dennis.co.uk
Printed in China.

Advertising
Katie Wood katie_wood@dennis.co.uk
Matt Wakefield matt_wakefield@dennis.co.uk

To subscribe to *Men's Fitness* magazine, call **0844 844 0081** or go to **www.mensfitness.co.uk**

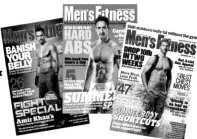

HAVE YOU GOT
WHAT IT TAKES TO

CHANGE?

Whether you are working towards your ideal physique in terms of appearance or whether you need your physique to deliver increased performance, you have a challenge on your hands.

Without maximizing each important component, you are likely to compromise or fail in your goals. When it comes to supplements, you might well need to change your views.

If you don't change your views, you may already have failed in your goals.

We've changed the industry standards of protein products for you.

We've changed what value for money can mean to you.

We've changed how products are formulated with you in mind.

We've changed how products are produced providing you with both performance and health.

We've changed the type of guarantee that you can expect.

We're totally committed to make changes to your physique and health more achievable.

Find out more about these changes at:

www.reflex-nutrition.com

 Please visit & join our Facebook page at Reflex Nutrition Ltd

 @ReflexNutrition

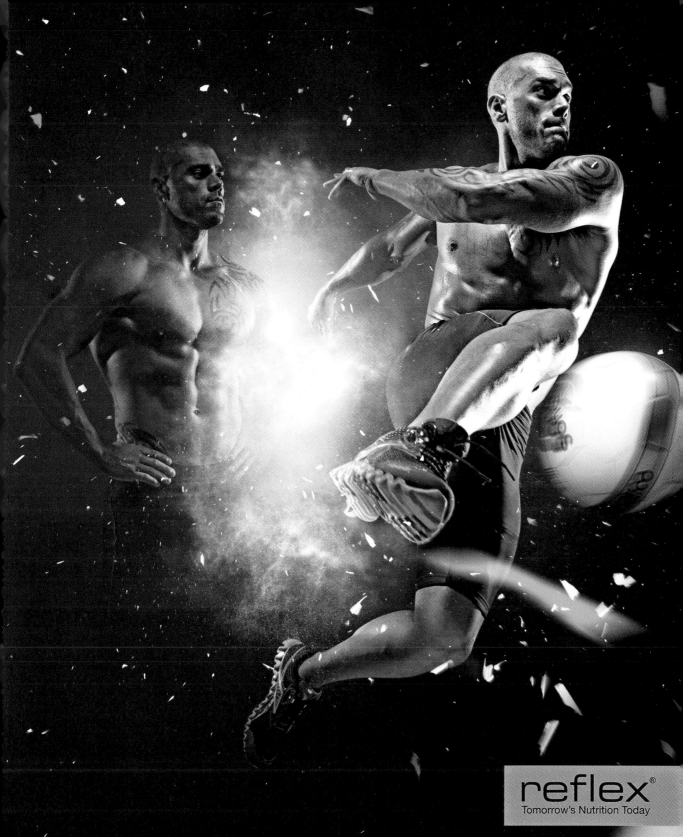

reflex®
Tomorrow's Nutrition Today

Men's Fitness ▶
Introduction

Welcome to the *Men's Fitness* Workout Manual, a collection of the best workouts and advice from the pages of Britain's finest fitness magazine.

The manual includes everything you need to get the body you've always wanted. The must-do moves section highlights the essential exercises that should form the foundation of your training. We've also created a six-month training plan and a nutrition section to give you easy-to-follow eating advice. The sports drills chapter gives you an insight into elite-level performance training while the abs moves section includes innovative moves that will help develop that coveted six-pack. And if you just want to trim a couple of inches off your waist the speedy fat-loss circuits in the final chapter will do just that.

Jon Lipsey, Editor, *Men's Fitness*

Contents

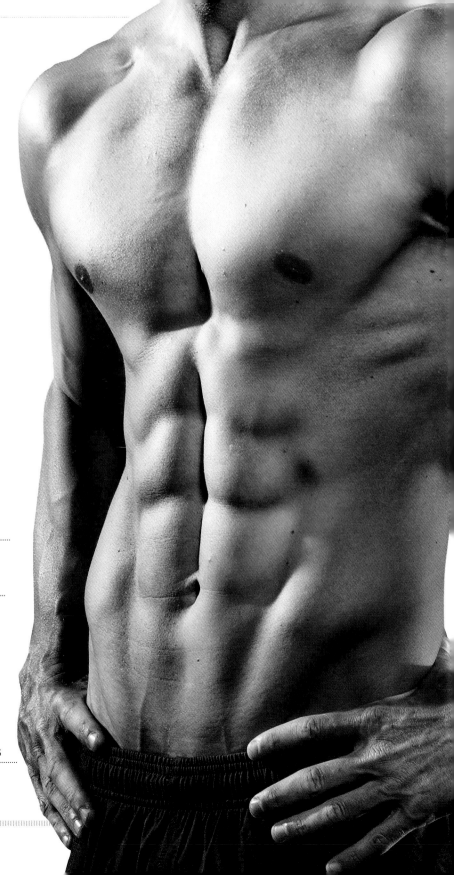

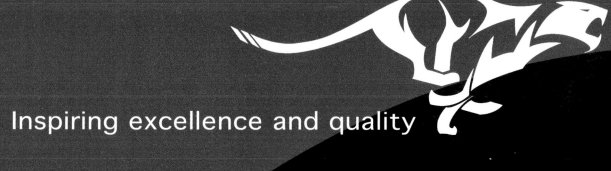

Inspiring excellence and quality

Steve Howarth
Natural World Bodybuilding Champion
Powered by EQ Nutrition
fueled by MM5

MM5 is the elite lean muscle builder by EQ Nutrition
Feed your body the five performance essentials

1.Protein
Lean muscle growth

2.Creatine
Power and explosive energy

3.Leucine
Ignition for lean growth

4.Glutamine
Muscle recovery

5.Taurine
Focus for the mind

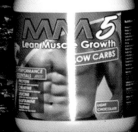

Order online for rapid next day delivery
Phone 01992 766 232

eqnutrition
eqnutrition.com

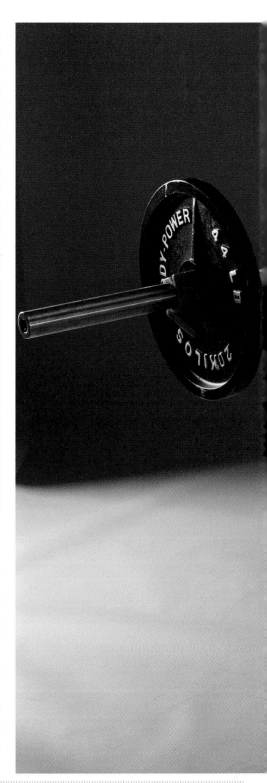

Must-do moves

These exercises are excellent at building muscle and burning fat. Here's how to get the most out of them

O ne of the biggest mistakes people make when they work out is favouring isolation moves such as biceps curls, which work one muscle group, over compound exercises such as the pull-up, which work multiple muscle groups.

The main reason for focusing on compound moves is that they recruit more muscle fibres than isolation moves. They also prompt the release of more of the hormones that are essential if you're looking to swap your gut for guns. By doing compound moves you also teach different body parts to work together, so you'll increase your stability and co-ordination and ultimately give your workouts bigger real-world benefits.

In this section we look at the key compound moves that you should include in your training programmes. We've also identified three or four assistance moves for each key lift, which you can work on to improve your performance in the big exercises.

KEY EXERCISES COVERED IN THIS SECTION

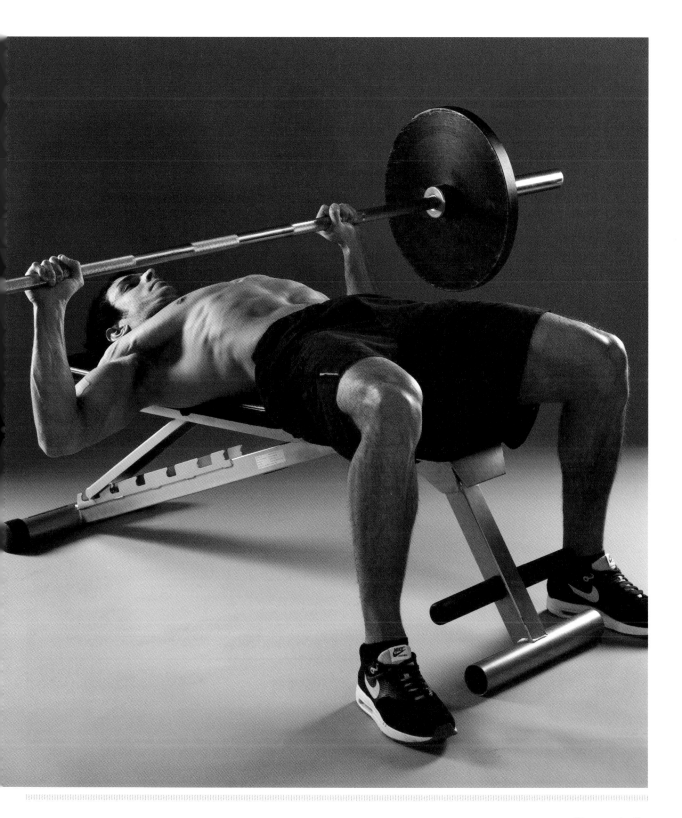

Deadlift

This classic move allows you to lift heavy and grow serious muscle – as long as you do it right. We show you how

The deadlift works wonders on your physique because it requires a team effort from lots of **muscles** and lets you load the bar heavy. To deadlift efficiently and safely you don't just need strong thighs and glutes – you should also improve the strength in your core, lower back and erector spinae, which supports and extends the spine. If you have an overdeveloped chest, it pulls you off-balance, and tight hamstrings don't allow you to adopt the necessary arch in the lower back. Here's how to do the lift and four smaller moves that will make sure you're strong in every part of the exercise.

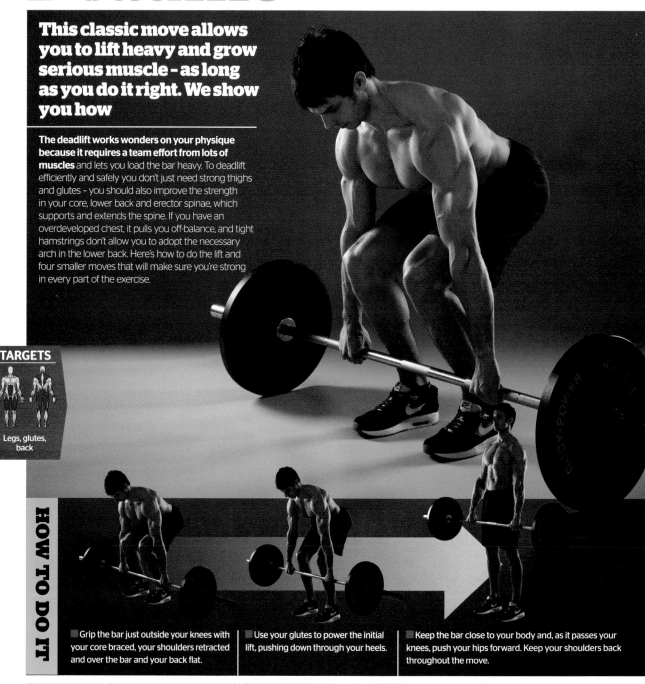

TARGETS

Legs, glutes, back

HOW TO DO IT

◾ Grip the bar just outside your knees with your core braced, your shoulders retracted and over the bar and your back flat.

◾ Use your glutes to power the initial lift, pushing down through your heels.

◾ Keep the bar close to your body and, as it passes your knees, push your hips forward. Keep your shoulders back throughout the move.

These moves will improve your deadlift

Single-leg Romanian deadlift

This move strengthens the glutes, hamstrings and lower back and targets the stabilising muscles in the supporting leg. This enables you to activate each glute independently, so when you return to two legs your stabilising muscles and glutes are switched on to provide you with a solid base.

How to do it
> Stand and hold the bar at arm's length with your feet shoulder-width apart.
> Keeping your knees soft, balance on one leg and lean your torso forwards until you feel a stretch in your hamstrings.
> Lift your torso again. Try to keep the bar off the floor for the entire set of reps.

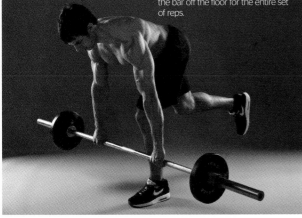

Bent-over row

An overdeveloped chest will pull you forward and knock you off balance when lifting. The pulling motion of the bent-over row strengthens your upper back and lats, which evens out your posture and puts you in a better position for a stronger lift, especially in the mid-shin phase when the bar wants to pull away from the body.

How to do it
> Start with your core braced, back straight and shoulders retracted. Lean forward from the hips and bend your knees slightly.
> Grip the bar with your hands just wider than shoulder-width apart, letting the bar hang at knee level.
> Pull the bar up to your sternum, squeezing your shoulder blades at the top, then lower slowly.

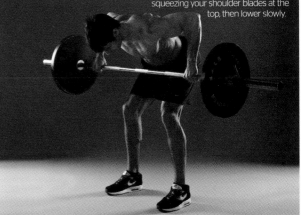

Sumo deadlift

The wider stance of the sumo deadlift recruits the glutes, one of the strongest muscles. It also stretches your adductors and helps you stay upright so you don't stress your hip flexors and lower back as much.

How to do it
> Stand behind the bar with your feet wider than shoulder-width apart and your toes pointing out. Squat down and grip the bar with your hands shoulder-width apart.
> Keeping your lower back in its natural arch, drive with your legs and push your hips forward, lifting the bar to your thighs.
> Reverse the motion, returning the bar to the floor.

Barbell suitcase deadlift

Because the weight is on one side, outside your centre of balance, your abs are going to be contracting hard to keep your torso vertical and stable as you come up with the bar. You are also going to be hitting your glutes, obliques and lats as you work each side of the body independently to stay upright. It will improve your grip strength too.

How to do it
> Place a barbell on your right side. Crouch down into a deadlift position and grab the bar with your right hand in the middle.
> Squeeze tight and deadlift the bar while keeping it level.

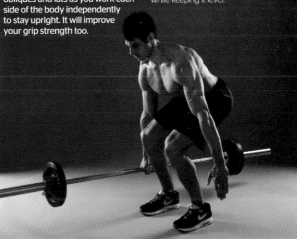

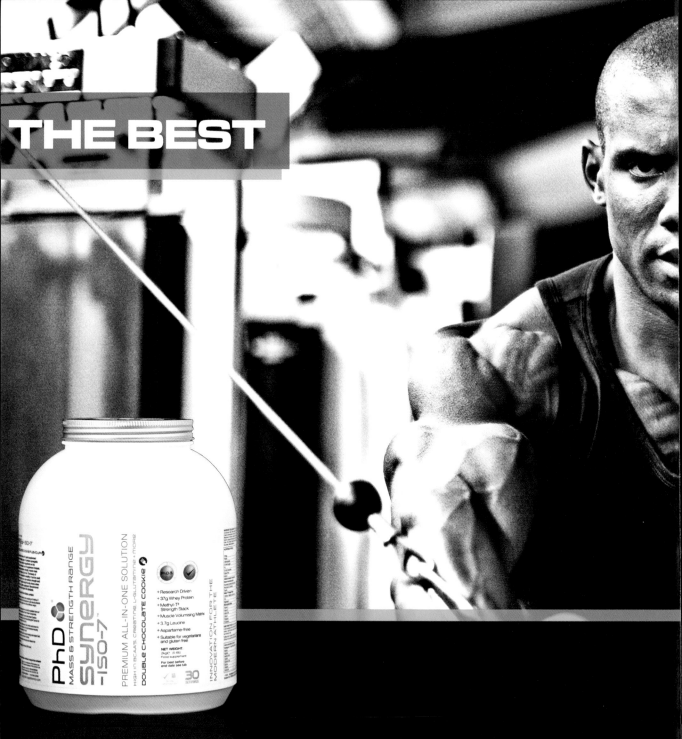

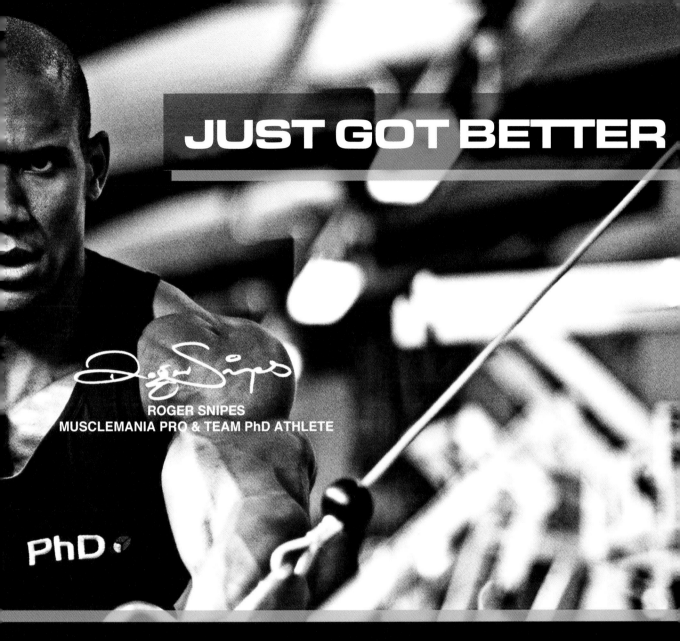

JUST GOT BETTER

ROGER SNIPES
MUSCLEMANIA PRO & TEAM PhD ATHLETE

PhD

NEW & IMPROVED FORMULA

Synergy-ISO-7 is the complete all-in-one sports nutrition product, containing over 35 grams of quality protein and a variety of added ingredients that ensures the serious athlete receives premium nutrition with each and every serving. Containing a powerful, strength-enhancing methyl-test stack, along with a triple action carbohydrate blend for energy and stamina, Synergy-ISO-7 now contains 5 grams of research proven Creatine Monohydrate per single serving and is perfect for all athletes seeking lean muscle, increased strength, fast recovery from intense training and improved performance. For a serious edge over your competitor, choose Synergy-ISO-7. Available from various national retailers, all good health stores and online web stores, in 2kg containers and 5 amazing PhD flavours.

Bench press

It's a classic indication of strength – but doing it wrong can lead to injury and bad posture

Your one-max rep on the bench press is a good indicator of upper body strength and gym dedication, so everyone wants an impressive score. The problem is that doing too much work on your chest and not enough on your back results in hunched shoulders, which in turn leads to a lack of range of motion and poor posture. It can also cause shoulder pain. You will need strong pecs, deltoids, lats and triceps for this lift..

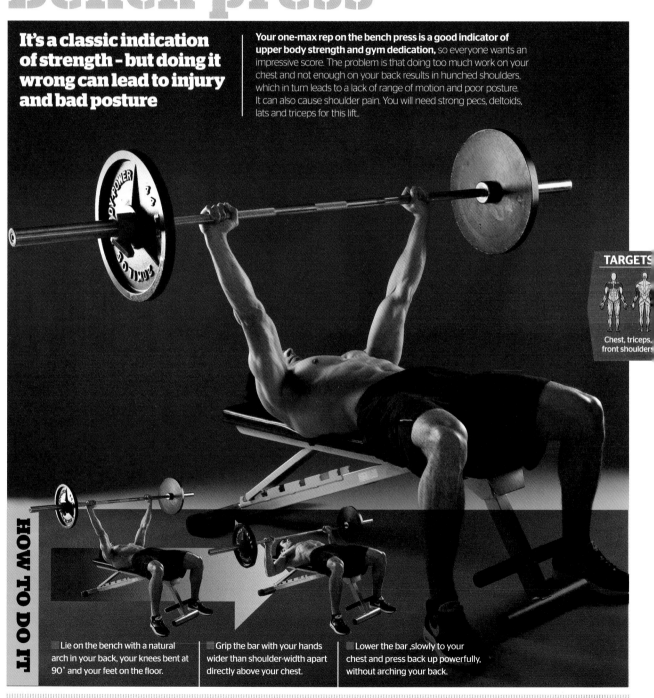

TARGETS

Chest, triceps, front shoulders

HOW TO DO IT

Lie on the bench with a natural arch in your back, your knees bent at 90° and your feet on the floor.

Grip the bar with your hands wider than shoulder-width apart directly above your chest.

Lower the bar ,slowly to your chest and press back up powerfully, without arching your back.

Four moves to boost your bench press

Serratus anterior pulse

With the support of the bench, the serratus anterior muscles – which run from the side of the chest to the shoulders – can get lazy when bench pressing, which restricts range of motion. This move will put your shoulders in the right position for the press.

How to do it
➤ Kneel with your hands on a gym ball, slightly wider than shoulder-width apart.
➤ Keeping your body in line, let your shoulder blades collapse inwards, then push them out while keeping your elbows straight and locked the whole time.

Spider-Man press-up

Many men think the bench press is the best exercise for the chest – but they're wrong. This move hits the chest but works the stabilising muscles around the shoulders too. It also hits the abs and lower back, which are often required to shift your weight in sports.

How to do it
➤ Get into a press-up position, then bend your elbows until your upper body is just off the floor, moving your right knee to your right elbow as you lower.
➤ Push up to the start using your chest, shoulders and triceps. Repeat on the other side.

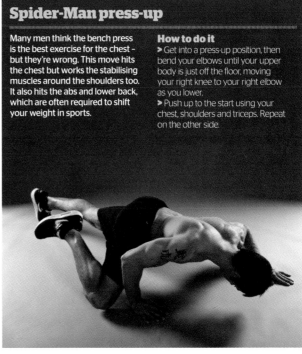

Incline one-arm press-up on step

The one-arm press-up requires immense strength and co-ordination between the chest, triceps, shoulder, glute and core muscles; all the muscles required for a strong bench press.

How to do it
➤ Place a step on the floor and get into a press-up position but with your right hand on the step.
➤ Perform a push-up.
➤ Repeat on the other side.

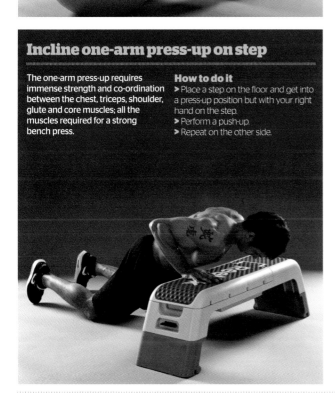

Medicine ball chest pass

The power aspect of this move kicks your nervous system into gear, while jump-starting your fast-twitch muscle fibres. This results in more responsive, stronger muscles, meaning you can use more weight on your lifts.

How to do it
➤ Stand with your feet shoulder-width apart and your core tight.
➤ Hold a medicine ball against your chest with both hands.
➤ Push with both hands to throw the ball against a wall or to a partner.

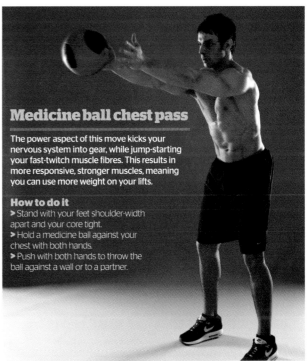

Squat

Strengthen your lower body so you can lift big weights without risking injury

Good squatting promotes balanced strength and a strong lower body, which is a great way to increase growth hormones around the body. But if you aren't lowering your body until your thighs are parallel to the floor or deeper, you're not completing the exercise's full range of motion. This is usually because of knee pain or placing too great a load on your lower back, so work the weak links for better gains. To do this, strengthen your knee joints and stretch your calves so your centre of gravity doesn't shift forward and place too much stress on your back. Then you'll be able to target the right muscles and get bigger and stronger. Follow this form guide to perfect your squat and, to lift more weight safely, do the moves opposite.

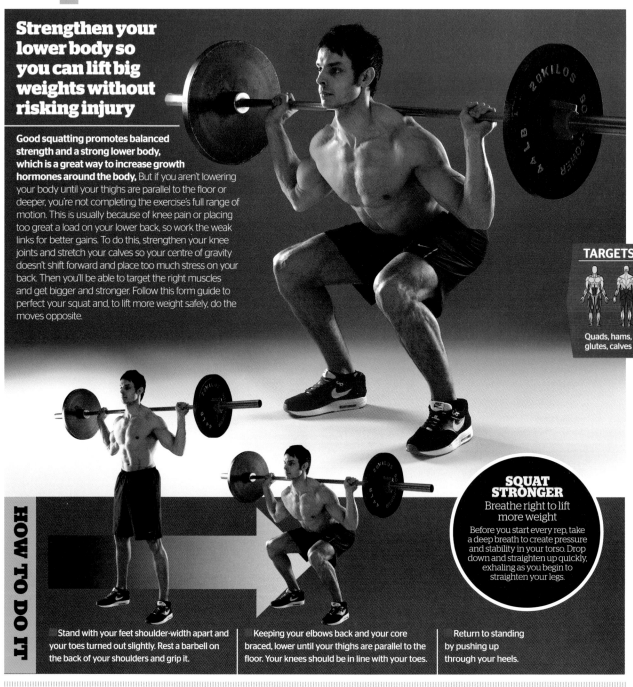

TARGETS

Quads, hams, glutes, calves

SQUAT STRONGER
Breathe right to lift more weight

Before you start every rep, take a deep breath to create pressure and stability in your torso. Drop down and straighten up quickly, exhaling as you begin to straighten your legs.

HOW TO DO IT

Stand with your feet shoulder-width apart and your toes turned out slightly. Rest a barbell on the back of your shoulders and grip it.

Keeping your elbows back and your core braced, lower until your thighs are parallel to the floor. Your knees should be in line with your toes.

Return to standing by pushing up through your heels.

One-legged decline squat

The decline forces your gluteus medius and quads to work harder, which stops the knee collapsing in as you squat and placing pressure on the joint. The decline also helps you develop strength and flexibility in your calves.

How to do it
➤ Set up a step on a slant. Stand on it facing the lower end.
➤ Balance on one leg, then bend your knee to squat as far as you can, keeping your back straight.
➤ Push up through your heel to the starting position.

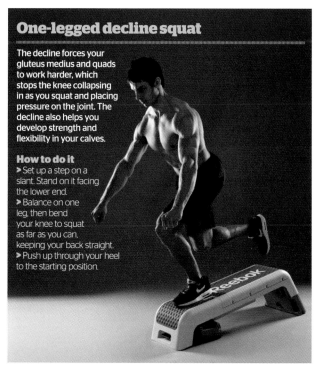

Wall slide

The wall slide is an excellent way to help you gain the functional control needed for a one-legged squat. It changes the angle of the squat, putting more emphasis on the gluteus medius, and helps strengthen the stabilising muscles in the ankle and knee.

How to do it
➤ Stand with your shoulder leaning against the wall. Lift the foot nearest the wall and get your balance.
➤ With your weight supported by the wall, bend your hips and knees and lower so that your thigh is parallel to the floor.
➤ Push back through your heel and straighten your leg to the start position.

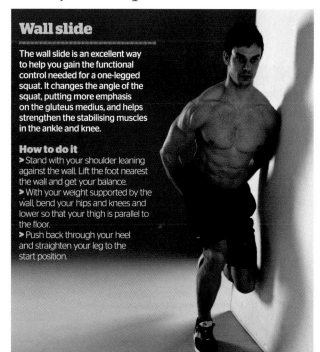

Knee and arm drive

Tight hip flexors will limit the flexibility in your quads and hamstrings, which limits your range of movement when doing a squat. They're shortened by too much sitting down so use this move to stretch them, so you can fire up the glutes and get more movement from your hamstrings.

How to do it
➤ Stand behind a box or platform. Place one foot on the platform with your heel close to the closest edge.
➤ Push off the box and drive your opposite knee up towards your chest.
➤ Repeat on the other leg.

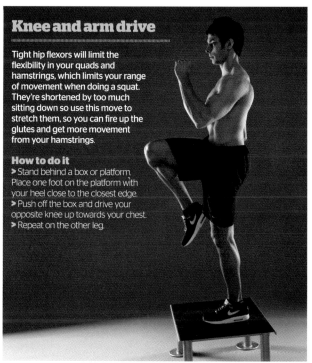

Squat jump

Explosive moves such as squat jumps recruit the maximum number of muscle fibres, which means that when you perform a normal squat you can lift more weight. It works by stimulating the nervous system, which makes your muscles ultra-responsive and prepared for a heavy load.

How to do it
➤ Stand with your feet shoulder-width apart and rest a light dumb-bell on each of your shoulders.
➤ With your elbows back and your core braced, lower until your thighs are parallel to the floor and then push up explosively to jump up.
➤ Land softly with your knees bent and lower into another squat.

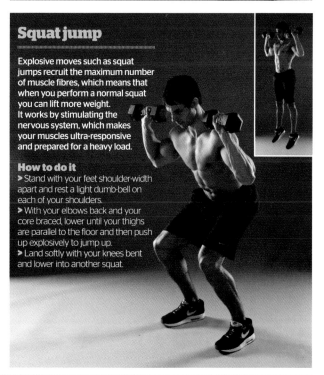

Bent-over row

It's a classic move for training your upper back, but the technique can be tricky. Here's how to do it right

The bent-over row works the opposite muscle group to the bench press – and the main difference is you provide your own platform using your lower body, core and glutes to support your weight. The key to the row is to retract your shoulder blades to allow the bar to come up to your chest, but too many men shrug their shoulders and round their back because they haven't got the strength in their traps, rhomboids and rear deltoids to control the movement. This takes the intended muscles out the equation and can cause imbalances. A strong core is also vital, because your upper back is worked the most when your torso is parallel to the floor, so your core will have to work hard to keep you stabilised.

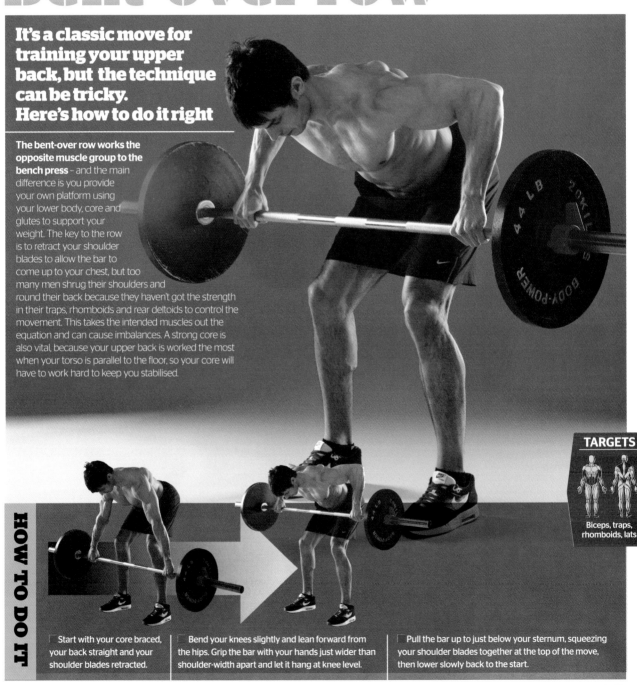

TARGETS

Biceps, traps, rhomboids, lats

HOW TO DO IT

☐ Start with your core braced, your back straight and your shoulder blades retracted.

☐ Bend your knees slightly and lean forward from the hips. Grip the bar with your hands just wider than shoulder-width apart and let it hang at knee level.

☐ Pull the bar up to just below your sternum, squeezing your shoulder blades together at the top of the move, then lower slowly back to the start.

These exercises will improve your bent-over row

Standing face pull with rotation

Face pulls improve posture and help build muscle in the upper back, especially your rotator cuff, rear deltoids and trapezius. Training these muscles not only helps you break through plateaus in almost every upper-body lift but also keeps your shoulders balanced and injuries at bay.

How to do it
➤ Stand in front of a cable station or resistance bands and grasp the handles with your palms facing the floor. Stand back so there is tension in the cables.
➤ Squeeze your shoulder blades together and pull the handles towards you until they're level with your face. Rotate your arms so your palms end up facing forward.
➤ Return to the starting position by allowing your arms to straighten out slowly in front of you.

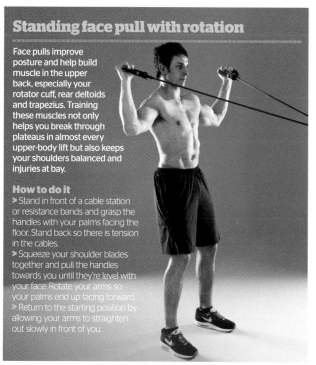

Gym ball T to cobra

This move strengthens the lower back and emphasises scapular retraction (pulling the shoulder blades back) by working the mid-traps and rhomboids. It also works your core, which has to work extra hard as you try to balance on the gym ball, while your posterior deltoids get a workout too.

How to do it
➤ Lie face down on a gym ball with your lower stomach resting on the ball and arms stretched above your heard.
➤ Raise your torso using the lower back, squeezing your glutes and keeping your head in line with your body.
➤ As you rise move your arms down to the sides of your body, squeezing your upper back.

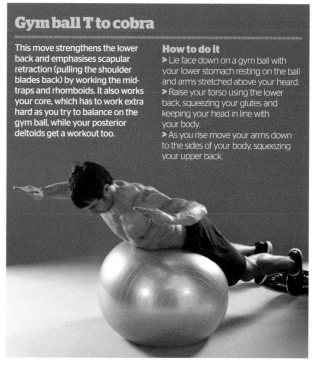

Renegade row

Pulling the weights from the floor discourages poor form because you can't use momentum to lift the weights up. Renegade rows also work your lats, deltoids, core strength and your horizontal pushing and pulling muscle groups.

How to do it
➤ Place a pair of dumb-bells on the floor shoulder-width apart and assume a press-up position over them with your body in a straight line from head to toe.
➤ Shift your weight to the left side of your body, and pull the right dumb-bell towards your hip in a rowing fashion. Return it to the floor slowly.
➤ Repeat on the other side.

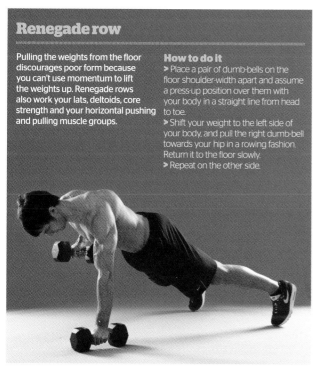

Inverted row

This move works all your major pulling muscles, but with even more emphasis on your core and lats. The inverted row will also correct bad posture and build your grip strength without putting any pressure on the lower back.

How to do it
➤ Set a horizontal bar at about chest height.
➤ Put your feet on a bench and lie underneath the bar holding it with an underhand grip, hands just wider than shoulder-width apart.
➤ Keeping your hips in line with your torso, pull your body up to the bar, trying to touch your sternum to it.
➤ Lower yourself slowly to the starting position.

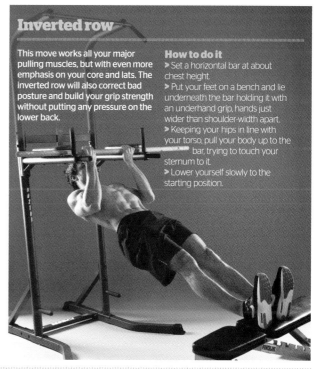

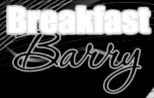
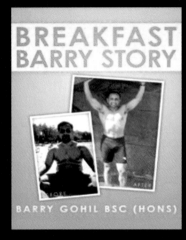

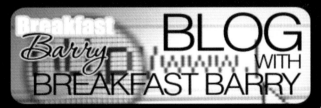
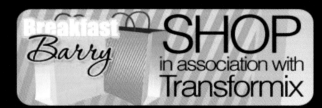
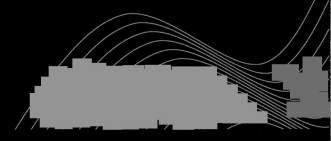

Pull-up

Raise your game with this upper-body muscle sculptor

The pull-up is one of the hardest lifts because you have to move your full bodyweight entirely and lift against gravity, which means the load on your muscles is very high. The advantage of this multi-tasking move is that it will balance the pushing work you're doing, so you don't get that hunched look. But if you don't already have the shoulder girdle, grip, forearm and lat [back] strength, you may struggle to do enough reps to get maximum strength gains. ▷

TARGETS

Biceps, traps, rhomboids, lats

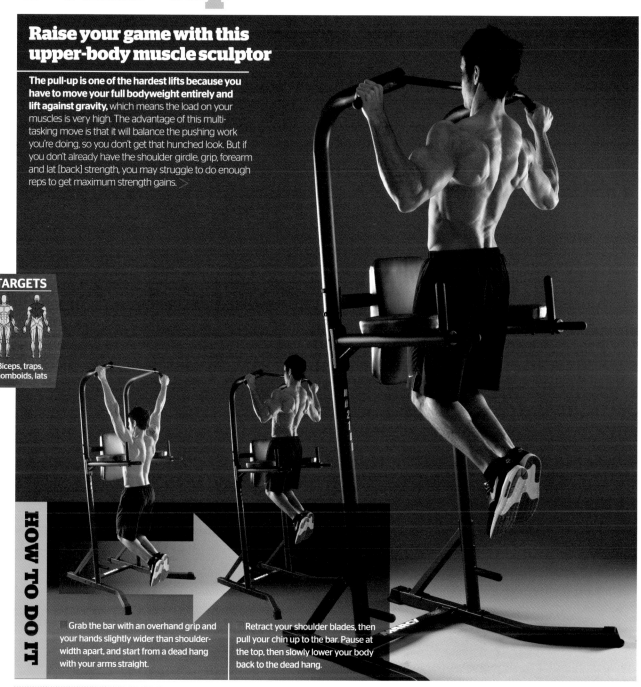

HOW TO DO IT

Grab the bar with an overhand grip and your hands slightly wider than shoulder-width apart, and start from a dead hang with your arms straight.

Retract your shoulder blades, then pull your chin up to the bar. Pause at the top, then slowly lower your body back to the dead hang.

Three moves to boost your pull-up

Bottoms-up kettlebell curl

This exercise strengthens your grip because a kettlebell is harder to hold than a dumb-bell. The increased difficulty will strengthen your biceps and forearms so they don't tire before your back muscles do, which means your back can get the workout you're trying to give it.

How to do it

> Grip the kettlebell tightly and draw the weight up the centre of your body with your elbow bent and close to your body. Keep the kettlebell in line with your forearm.
> Squeeze the handle tightly, engage your core muscles and slowly lower the bell back down to your thigh.
> Once the bell is lowered, pause before curling it back to the start.

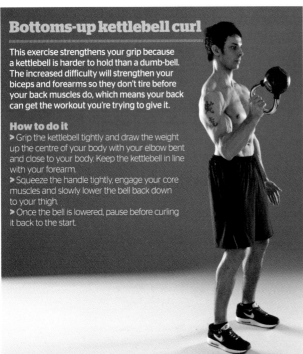

Trap depression

This increases your range of motion in your joints and flexibility in your large muscle groups. This helps your lower traps because compromised mobility from tight muscles impedes growth.

How to do it

> Start like you're doing a dip, with straight arms, upper body upright and chest out.
> Push your shoulders and arms downwards, making sure you keep the arms straight throughout the move and focusing on using the lower traps.
> Slowly shrug your shoulders and arms upwards to your ears.

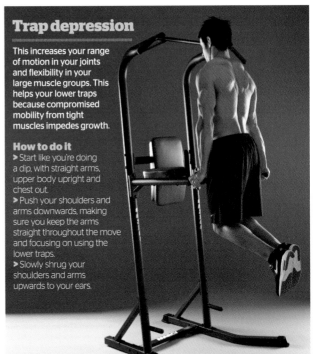

Bent-over row

An overdeveloped chest will pull you forward and knock you off balance when lifting. The pulling motion of the bent-over row strengthens your upper back and lats, which evens out your posture and puts you in a better position for a stronger lift, especially in the mid-shin phase when the bar wants to pull away from the body.

How to do it

> Start with your core braced, back straight and shoulders retracted. Lean forward from the hips and bend your knees.
> Grip the bar just wider than shoulder-width apart, letting the bar hang at knee level.
> Pull the bar up to your sternum, squeezing your shoulder blades at the top, then lower slowly.

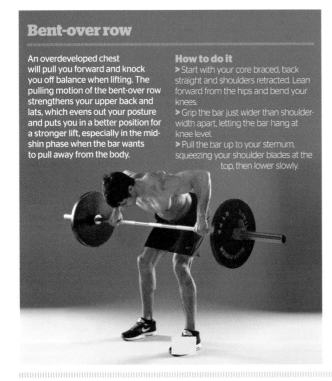

Full-range dumb-bell biceps curl uppercut

The point of this exercise is to work the biceps through a larger range of motion. This will develop strength along the full length of the biceps muscles, ultimately giving greater strength gains.

How to do it

> Holding a dumb-bell, begin a biceps curl.
> When your elbow gets to 90°, start to perform an uppercut-style action with the knuckles going up to the ceiling and arm lifting. Let your body rotate and foot swivel as if you were uppercut punching.
> Pause at the top and reverse the move under control, still using the biceps to control the weight.

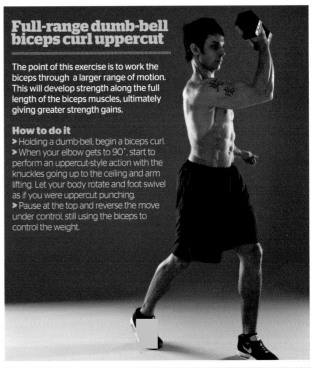

DECLARE WAR ON FAT

LET BATTLE COMMENCE!

- **Multi award winning fatburner and the world's fastest growing weight loss brand, sold in over 130 countries**
- **Advanced thermogenic formula designed to suppress appetite and increase energy**
- **Contains key ingredients clinically proven to burn fat and support weight loss**
- **Used by professional athletes, fitness enthusiasts, military personnel and Special Forces worldwide**

1 day trial packs now available at selected stores

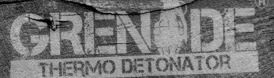

Must-Do Moves

Lunge

Build strong, powerful legs with this classic muscle move

'When building strong legs most people overlook lunges in favour of squats,' but lunging is a basic movement pattern that requires power and co-ordination, both of which are vital for sports,' says Neil Odell, a personal trainer and founder of Fit For My Day (fit4myday. com). 'Lunges work the powerhouse lower-body muscles, such as the glutes, quads, hamstrings and calves, but also involve the adductors, hip flexors and many other stabilising muscles – including your core – that need to be strong to allow you to move with speed and power.'

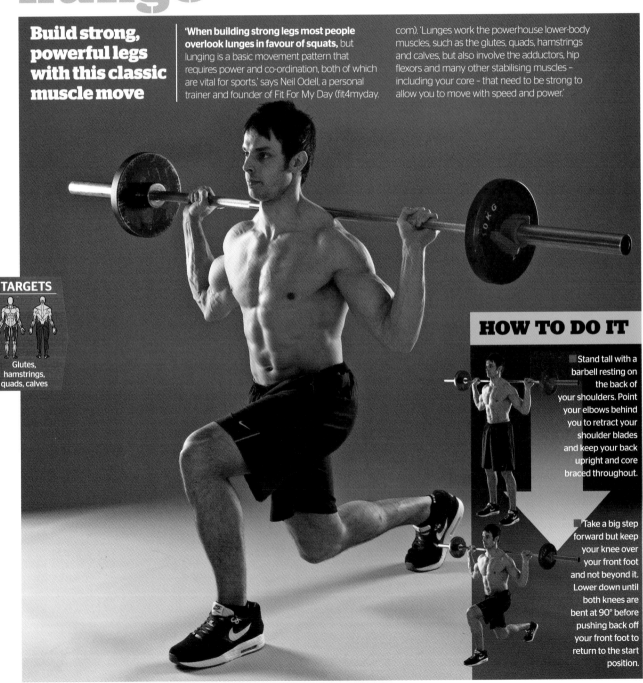

TARGETS

Glutes, hamstrings, quads, calves

HOW TO DO IT

■ Stand tall with a barbell resting on the back of your shoulders. Point your elbows behind you to retract your shoulder blades and keep your back upright and core braced throughout.

■ Take a big step forward but keep your knee over your front foot and not beyond it. Lower down until both knees are bent at 90° before pushing back off your front foot to return to the start position.

Four moves to improve your lunge

Wall slide

This is a great move to target the smaller muscles of the glutes, which play a vital role in keeping your leg in a strong and stable position during one-leg moves such as the lunge.

How to do it
> Lean against the wall and raise one foot off the ground.
> Slowly lower yourself down as far as is comfortable before slowing pushing back up on your standing leg to return to the start position.

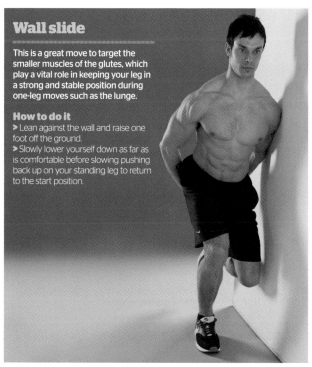

Lunge and twist with band

This progression from a basic lunge places emphasis on your core muscles, especially the obliques, and is a great move to improve your ability to lunge and turn at speed when playing sport.

How to do it
> Attach a resistance band to a fixed object next to you.
> Holding the other end of the band in your hands, lunge forward and rotate your torso away from the object.
> Twist back as you return to the start position. Repeat each side.

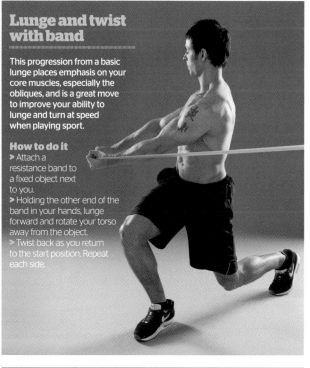

Split squat bar between legs

If you have poor posture because of tightness in your back muscles and struggle to maintain a load on your back, this exercise can improve your ability to lunge and build strength to progress on to harder moves.

How to do it
> Stand in a split stance with one foot in front of a barbell and the other behind it.
> Holding the barbell with your hands out by your sides, lunge down and up, lifting the barbell with each rep.

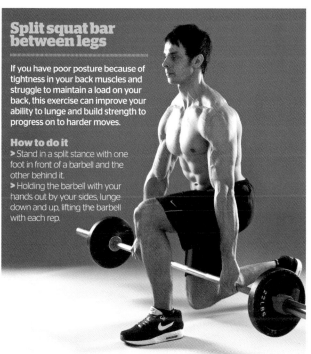

Curtsy squat

Another great move for sportsmen, because it works the stabilising muscles of your core, hips and legs, allowing you to move more powerfully and under control on the field. You'll also be able to lift more weight during lunges thanks to better support from these stronger stabilising muscles.

How to do it
> Start with your feet hip-width apart.
> Take a big step forward with one leg but instead of going straight out in front, swing your leg out and across your back leg before lunging down until both knees are bent at 90°.
> Return slowly to the start.

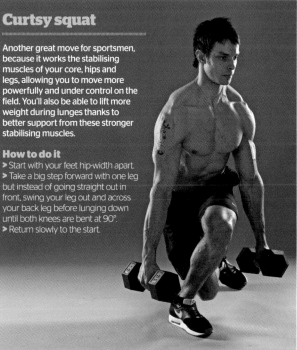

Must-Do Moves

Triceps dip

Build big arms with this classic bodyweight move

When building big arms, a lot of guys favour biceps moves over those exercises that focus on the triceps. But the triceps make up about two-thirds of your upper-arm musculature, so you can't afford to ignore this muscle if you want to add some size and strength. Dips are also great for working the lower chest and shoulders, especially the small, stabilising muscles of the shoulder joint that get neglected when using resistance machines, and your core, which you must keep tight to prevent your lower body from swinging.

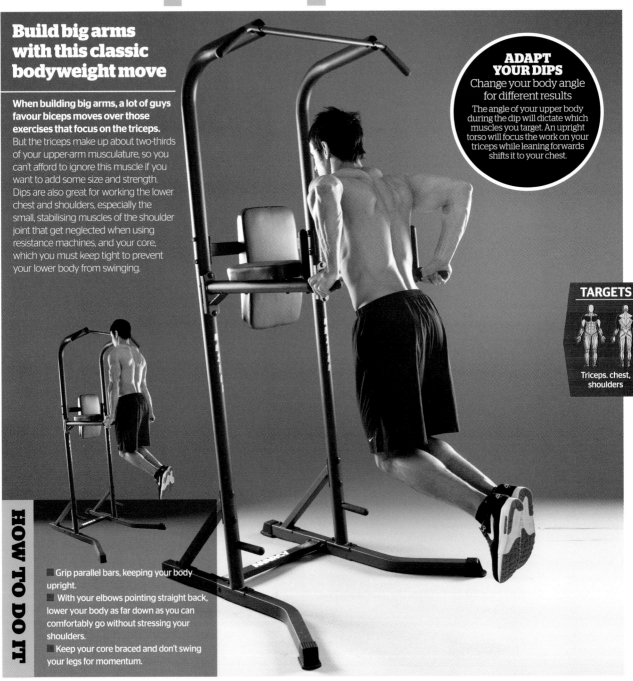

ADAPT YOUR DIPS
Change your body angle for different results
The angle of your upper body during the dip will dictate which muscles you target. An upright torso will focus the work on your triceps while leaning forwards shifts it to your chest.

TARGETS
Triceps, chest, shoulders

HOW TO DO IT

◼ Grip parallel bars, keeping your body upright.

◼ With your elbows pointing straight back, lower your body as far down as you can comfortably go without stressing your shoulders.

◼ Keep your core braced and don't swing your legs for momentum.

Dip bar raise

This is a great move for improving shoulder strength and stability, as well as working your upper back.

How to do it

> Grip parallel bars and support your bodyweight on your arms.
> Keeping your arms straight, push yourself up by squeezing your shoulder blades together.
> Keep your chest up and your core braced.

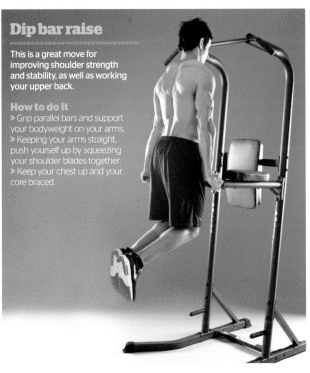

T press-up

This twist on the classic move requires greater upper-body co-ordination, strong triceps to support your bodyweight and a strong core to rotate upwards.

How to do it

> Start in a press-up position and lower your chest to the ground, keeping your elbows close to your side.
> Press back up powerfully and at the top of the move, lift one arm off the ground while twisting your torso until that arm is pointing towards the ceiling.
> Lower back down before repeating the other side.

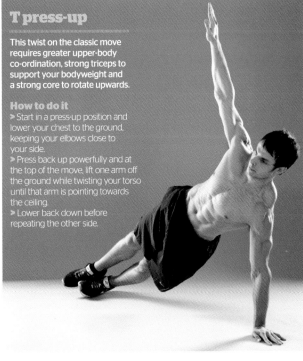

Medicine ball press-up

This press-up variation places greater emphasis on the triceps, while the instability of the ball forces your core to work overtime to keep your body rigid.

How to do it

> Start in a press-up position but with your hands either side of a medicine ball, rather than flat on the floor.
> Keeping your body in a straight line from head to heels, lower until your chest touches the ball before powering back up strongly.

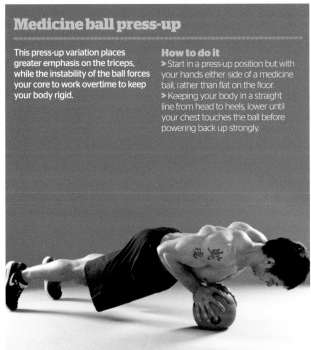

Lying triceps extension

This move isolates your triceps muscles, forcing them to work hard throughout the entire move.

How to do it

> Lie flat on a bench, holding dumb-bells above you with your arms kept straight.
> Slowly lower the weights towards the top of your head by bending your elbows, which should stay pointing directly to the ceiling.
> Without arching your back, slowly return the dumb-bells to the start position by straightening your arms.

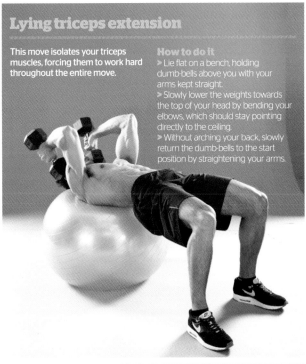

Hang clean

Master this monster move to get stronger and bigger

The hang clean is a great total-body exercise that develops strength and power because you have to perform the move fast in order to move the weight from the floor to your shoulders. This makes it a fantastic exercise to do if you want to build power for sport or improve your performance at other big moves, especially squats and deadlifts. If you have hit a plateau and want to shake things up, it's suitably tough as a new exercise. And because it gets your heart pumping fast, it's also great for increasing your metabolism so you burn more fat.

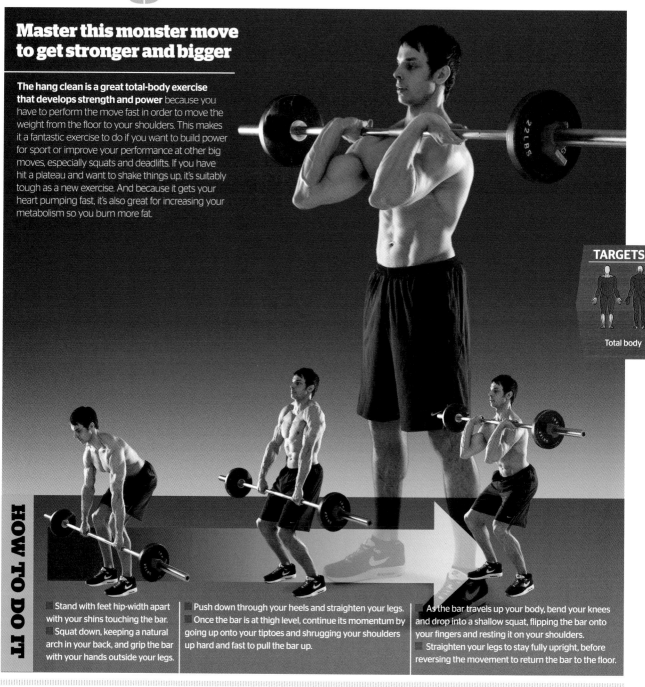

TARGETS

Total body

HOW TO DO IT

■ Stand with feet hip-width apart with your shins touching the bar.
■ Squat down, keeping a natural arch in your back, and grip the bar with your hands outside your legs.

■ Push down through your heels and straighten your legs.
■ Once the bar is at thigh level, continue its momentum by going up onto your tiptoes and shrugging your shoulders up hard and fast to pull the bar up.

■ As the bar travels up your body, bend your knees and drop into a shallow squat, flipping the bar onto your fingers and resting it on your shoulders.
■ Straighten your legs to stay fully upright, before reversing the movement to return the bar to the floor.

Three moves to improve your hang clean

Squat to calf raise

This is a great move for getting to grips with the first part of the hang clean and developing the power you need to get the move started.

How to do it

> Start in a squat position with knees over your toes, back in a natural arch and chest high.

> Drive upwards through your heels, before pushing your hips forward.
> As your legs begin to straighten, rise up on the tips of your toes.
> Keep your core braced throughout.

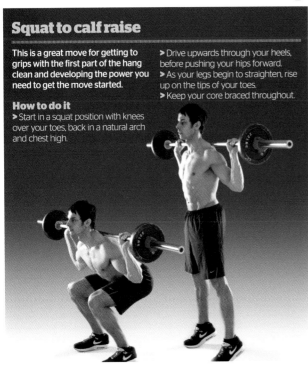

Dumb-bell lunge and rotate

Without a strong core you can't efficiently transfer power from your lower to upper body, so this move works on core strength in addition to improving co-ordination.

How to do it

> Start by holding a dumb-bell in both hands above your head.
> Take a step forwards and lower until both knees are bent at 90°, keeping your torso upright.
> As you lunge, lower the weight down and across your leading leg, then push through your front footto return to the start.

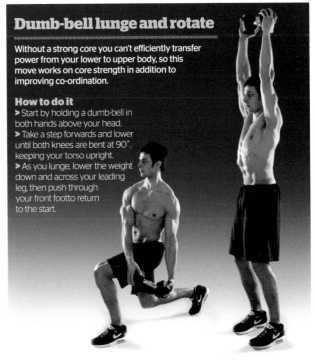

Dumb-bell high pull

This move will help you improve the second part of the move, the one that most people find the hardest to get right, by testing your ability to transfer power from your lower to upper body. Using dumb-bells makes the move more manageable and will improve strength and co-ordination to progress to a barbell.

How to do it

> Start in a wide split stance, holding a dumb-bell by your front foot.
> Drive upwards through your heels and push your hips forward while shrugging your shoulders to generate power to lift the dumb-bell higher.

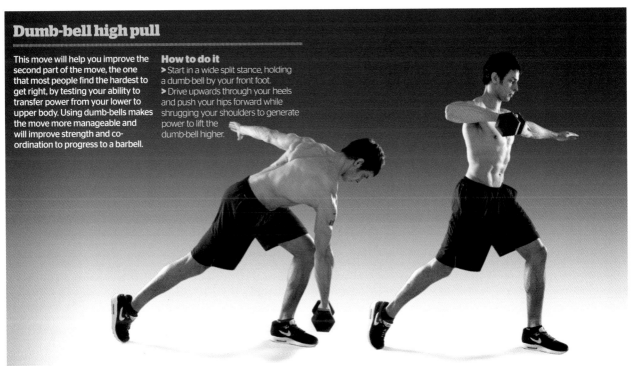

Snatch

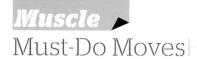

This is an effective whole-body muscle-building lift and nothing else

This Olympic lift builds flexibility and co-ordination as well as muscle. Commonly linked to powerlifting, this posterior chain move improves explosive movement, strength, speed and core stability. Numerous sports mimic its movement pattern in some form – for example, lifting a rugby player in the lineout. As with all big lifts, you need to ensure you set up correctly and focus your mind completely on the lift to get it right. This is a tricky move so do it using a light bar to perfect your form before you start lifting serious weight.

TARGETS

Whole body

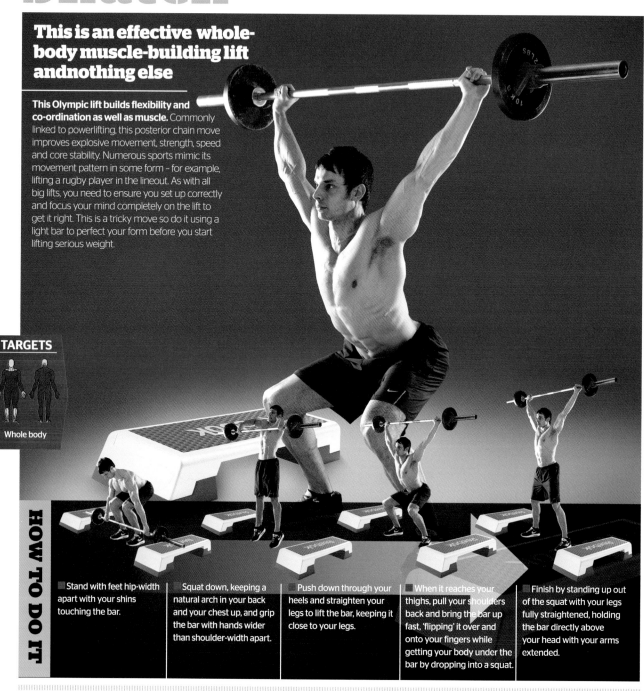

HOW TO DO IT

■ Stand with feet hip-width apart with your shins touching the bar.

■ Squat down, keeping a natural arch in your back and your chest up, and grip the bar with hands wider than shoulder-width apart.

■ Push down through your heels and straighten your legs to lift the bar, keeping it close to your legs.

■ When it reaches your thighs, pull your shoulders back and bring the bar up fast, 'flipping' it over and onto your fingers while getting your body under the bar by dropping into a squat.

■ Finish by standing up out of the squat with your legs fully straightened, holding the bar directly above your head with your arms extended.

Four moves to boost your snatch

Medicine ball overhead lunge to bend

Increasing the strength and stability of your core, upper body and legs, this is the perfect way to improve your snatch form.

How to do it
> Stand with one leg in front of the other while holding a medicine ball at arm's length.
> Bend over from the waist and then swing the ball upwards above your head.
> As you swing upwards, lunge forward with your legs. Hold the stance when your arms are fully extended.
> Return to the starting position and repeat, lunging with the other leg.

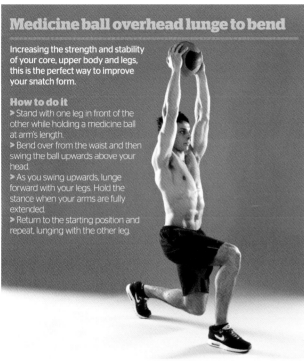

Calf foam roller

When lifting a heavy weight above your head, you need to make sure that every muscle is able to take the strain and stay stable. The foam roller is a great way to add a layer of support to your calf muscles and give them the extra strength they need when performing a snatch.

How to do it
> Get a foam roller and put it under your calves.
> Lift your body off the floor using your hands and, with your toes pointed out, slowly move the roller from your calf to your knee.
> Repeat as necessary or do it with one leg at a time to increase the difficulty.

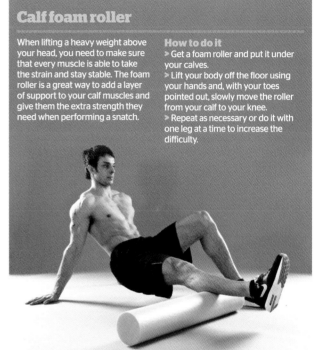

Thoracic rotation

To increase the weight on your snatch, you need good mobility, posture and technique as well as strength. This move will help in this, as well as reducing the pressure on your back and shoulders.

How to do it
> Secure a stretch band to something solid and stand next to it with one foot in front of the other and both legs bent at the knee slightly.
> Grasp the band with both hands and pull it across your body.
> As you pull, twist your torso against the resistance before slowly returning to the starting position.
> Be sure to work both sides of your body.

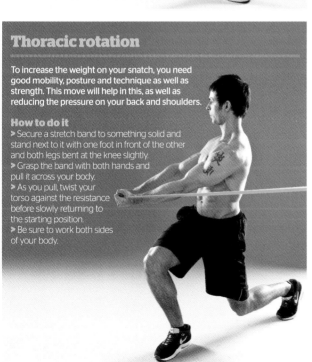

Kettlebell clean

Whether you're a beginner or an expert, you can never work on your form too much. This move will increase your strength and stability as well as improve your clean technique.

How to do it
> Hold a kettlebell by your side and keep your back straight and chest out.
> Push the kettlebell between your legs before driving your arm forward, using your core, hips and legs to lift the weight and flip it over onto the front of your shoulder.
> Slowly return to the start then repeat the move, using the downward momentum get the next rep started.

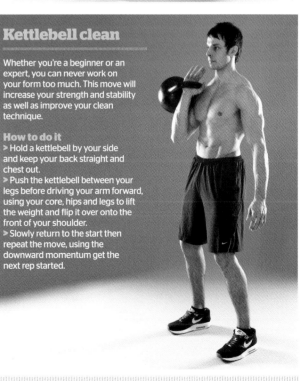

Must-Do Moves

Clean and press

No, don't get the ironing board out – instead master this often-ignored classic lift to reap total-body benefits

This is an exercise that every guy should do, but many don't because of its complexity. It requires every major muscle group to work together efficiently in order to lift the bar from the floor to over your head. Get this exercise right and you'll build strength and stability from top to toe and improve explosive power, which has a great crossover to many sports.

Because it involves so many muscles, this is a high-risk move so it is best to start with a light barbell and master the correct form before adding additional weight. It also puts pressure on your lower back, so build strength there with the squat, deadlift and overhead press and you'll improve your progress.

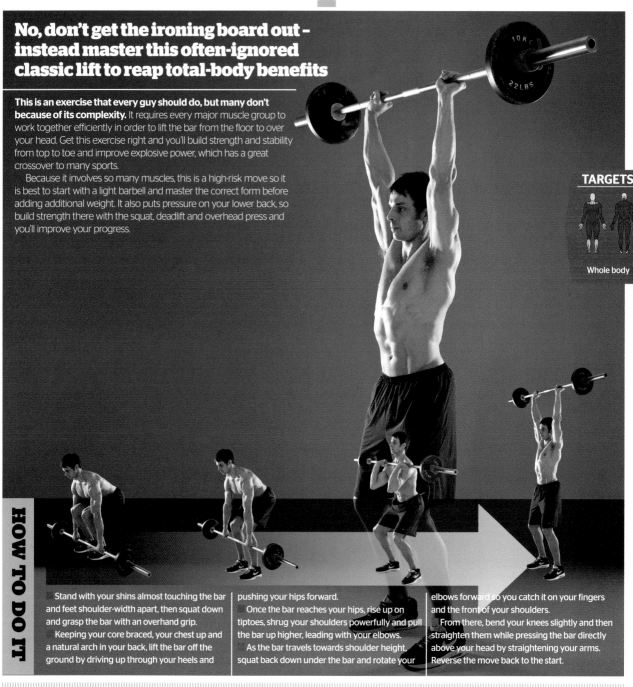

TARGETS

Whole body

HOW TO DO IT

Stand with your shins almost touching the bar and feet shoulder-width apart, then squat down and grasp the bar with an overhand grip.

Keeping your core braced, your chest up and a natural arch in your back, lift the bar off the ground by driving up through your heels and pushing your hips forward.

Once the bar reaches your hips, rise up on tiptoes, shrug your shoulders powerfully and pull the bar up higher, leading with your elbows.

As the bar travels towards shoulder height, squat back down under the bar and rotate your elbows forward so you catch it on your fingers and the front of your shoulders.

From there, bend your knees slightly and then straighten them while pressing the bar directly above your head by straightening your arms. Reverse the move back to the start.

Four moves to improve your clean and press

Single-leg deadlift to shoulder press

Form and stability are key to the clean and press so performing this exercise on only one leg will both strengthen your core and force you to concentrate on technique. When it's time for the actual lift, you'll feel far more confident.

How to do it
> Hold a dumb-bell in one hand and stand on one foot.
> Bend at the hips so you lower the weight almost to the floor, keeping your back straight.
> Slowly straighten up and pull the dumb-bell up in front of you before 'flipping' the weight onto your upturned palm and pressing it overhead.
> Switch legs and arms and repeat.

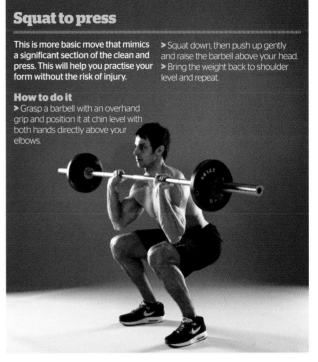

Squat to press

This is more basic move that mimics a significant section of the clean and press. This will help you practise your form without the risk of injury.

How to do it
> Grasp a barbell with an overhand grip and position it at chin level with both hands directly above your elbows.
> Squat down, then push up gently and raise the barbell above your head.
> Bring the weight back to shoulder level and repeat.

Multi-planar lunge to press

The pressing movement of this exercise will again prepare your body for the upper part of the lift, while the lunges put the spotlight on your legs and core.

How to do it
> Hold a dumb-bell in each hand and raise them to shoulder level.
> Lunge forward with your left leg, pressing the weights as you return to a standing position.
> Repeat this technique with the right leg, then lunge to both sides as well as doing a standing turn lunge, stepping back at a 45° angle alternately with your left and right foot.
> Remember to press the dumb-bells overhead between each lunge.

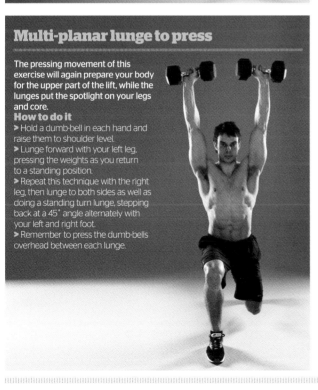

Kettlebell clean

Because the weight is on one side, outside your centre of balance, your abs are going to be contracting hard to keep your torso vertical and stable as you come up with the bar. You are also going to be hitting your glutes, obliques and lats as you work each side of the body independently to stay upright. It will improve your grip strength too.

How to do it
> Place a barbell on your right side. Crouch down into a deadlift position and grab the bar with your right hand in the middle.
> Squeeze tight and deadlift the bar while keeping it level.

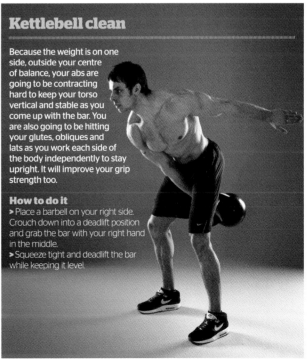

Shoulder press

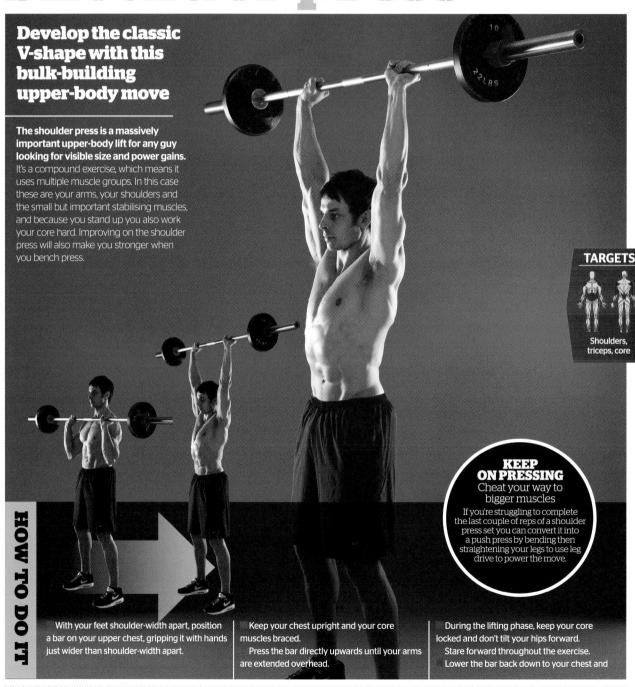

Develop the classic V-shape with this bulk-building upper-body move

The shoulder press is a massively important upper-body lift for any guy looking for visible size and power gains. It's a compound exercise, which means it uses multiple muscle groups. In this case these are your arms, your shoulders and the small but important stabilising muscles, and because you stand up you also work your core hard. Improving on the shoulder press will also make you stronger when you bench press.

TARGETS

Shoulders, triceps, core

KEEP ON PRESSING
Cheat your way to bigger muscles

If you're struggling to complete the last couple of reps of a shoulder press set you can convert it into a push press by bending then straightening your legs to use leg drive to power the move.

HOW TO DO IT

With your feet shoulder-width apart, position a bar on your upper chest, gripping it with hands just wider than shoulder-width apart.

Keep your chest upright and your core muscles braced.
Press the bar directly upwards until your arms are extended overhead.

During the lifting phase, keep your core locked and don't tilt your hips forward.
Stare forward throughout the exercise.
Lower the bar back down to your chest and

Three moves to boost your shoulder press

Gym ball row and rotation

This exercise hits your rotator cuff muscles. If these are strong you'll be able to lift far more weight in the shoulder press.

How to do it
> Lie with your chest on a gym ball with a dumb-bell in each hand.
> Lift the weights until your forearms are at 90° to your head, with your palms facing downwards.
> Keeping your upper arms still, rotate your arms to raise the weights until they're level with your head.

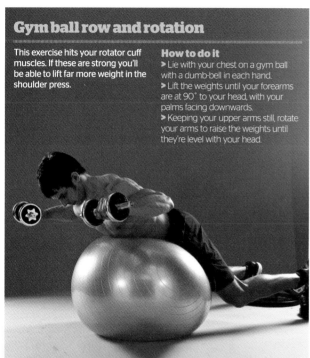

One-arm standing kettlebell press

Using a kettlebell, with its uneven weight distribution, causes greater engagement of your core muscles as you try to counter-balance the shifting load. Stronger core muscles will enable you to lift more on a wide range of exercises.

How to do it
> Hold a kettlebell in front of your chest, with your palm facing your chest and your arm tucked in to your body.
> Contract your abs, glutes and lats to improve your stability.
> Press the kettlebell up by extending your elbow and rotate your arm so your palm faces forward.
> Keep your forearm vertical as you raise and lower the kettlebell.

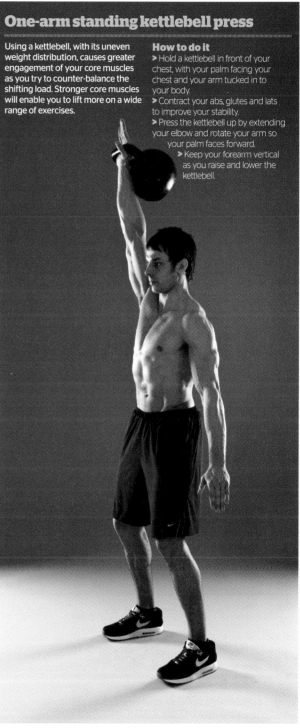

Prone shoulder press

This beginner-friendly move targets the rear deltoids and traps, making it a great move to develop the muscles involved in the shoulder press.

How to do it
> Lie with your core on a gym ball with a dumb-bell in each hand.
> Raise your arms so your hands are level with your head and your elbows are bent at 90°.
> Extend your arms out and in front of you, pause briefly, then slowly return to the start.

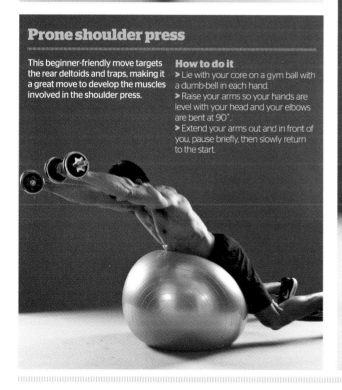

Must-Do Moves

Kettlebell swing

If you want a hardcore total-body move that will build muscle and burn fat, put the kettle on

The two-handed kettlebell swing is an efficient way to build power in the posterior chain muscles, including the glutes and hamstrings, which is essential for any sport that requires explosive movement. You'll improve your strength but you'll also feel your heart rate soaring and get a great cardio workout too, because this is a high-intensity exercise that will fire up your fat-burning furnace. As a functional exercise it will also have the knock-on effect of building integrity in your lower spine, making everyday tasks easier to perform and reducing your risk of injury.

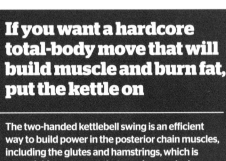

TARGETS

Glutes, hamstrings, shoulders, lower back, core

HOW TO DO IT

■ With your feet shoulder-width apart, hold a kettlebell in both hands.
■ Keeping your back straight and your knees in line with your feet, squat at the hips and swing the kettlebell in a controlled way between your legs.
■ Brace your core, then stand up and snap your hips forward to propel the kettlebell forwards and upwards to shoulder height. The power should come from your hips, not your arms.
■ Continue the swing in a fluid, controlled movement.

SWING THOSE HIPS

Hinge at the hips to avoid injury

Most people instinctively bend their knees when doing kettlebell swings but the key is to hinge at the hips and keep your knees relatively straight. Make sure you really drive with your hips with each swing.

Glute bridge

This will help you to swing the kettlebell better by targeting your core, glutes and hamstrings in a compound movement. 'This is an ideal preparation for the swing, especially if you haven't used kettlebells before,' says Hodgkin.

How to do it
➤ Lie with your back and hips on the floor and your knees bent.
➤ Keep your feet flat on the floor and your arms by your sides.
➤ Tighten your stomach muscles and raise your hips until your body is in a straight line from your shoulders to your knees.
➤ Hold for 20 seconds, then lower, pause and repeat.

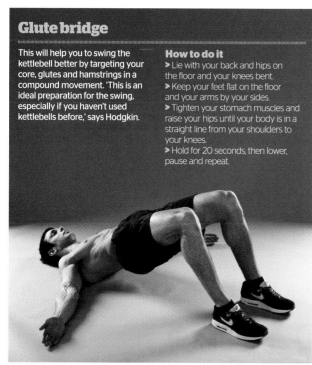

One-arm swing

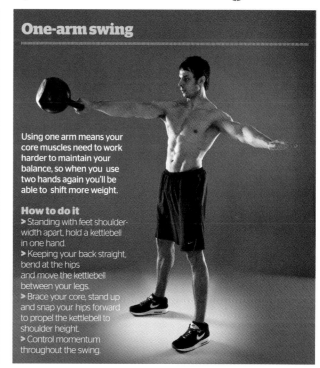

Using one arm means your core muscles need to work harder to maintain your balance, so when you use two hands again you'll be able to shift more weight.

How to do it
➤ Standing with feet shoulder-width apart, hold a kettlebell in one hand.
➤ Keeping your back straight, bend at the hips and move the kettlebell between your legs.
➤ Brace your core, stand up and snap your hips forward to propel the kettlebell to shoulder height.
➤ Control momentum throughout the swing.

Towel swing

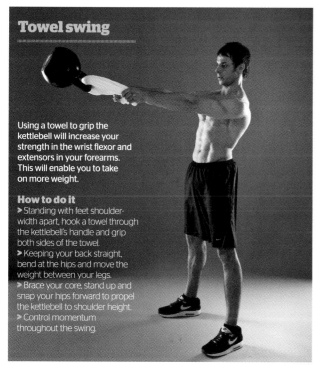

Using a towel to grip the kettlebell will increase your strength in the wrist flexor and extensors in your forearms. This will enable you to take on more weight.

How to do it
➤ Standing with feet shoulder-width apart, hook a towel through the kettlebell's handle and grip both sides of the towel.
➤ Keeping your back straight, bend at the hips and move the weight between your legs.
➤ Brace your core, stand up and snap your hips forward to propel the kettlebell to shoulder height.
➤ Control momentum throughout the swing.

Box jump

Jumps are a plyometric exercise which develop the ability to recruit large numbers of muscle fibres quickly in the lower body. 'That's exactly what you need to powerfully swing a kettlebell,' says Hodgkin.

How to do it
➤ Stand in front of a bench or box.
➤ With your feet shoulder-width apart, squat down and explosively jump up onto the box.
➤ Step back down and repeat.

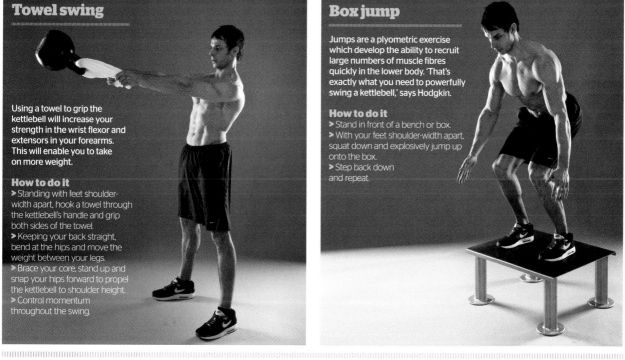

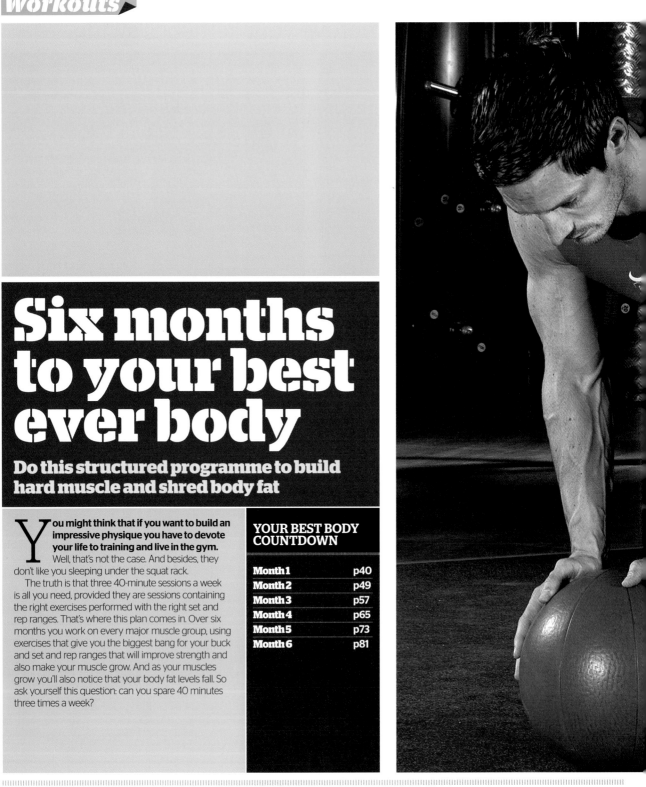

Six months to your best ever body

Do this structured programme to build hard muscle and shred body fat

You might think that if you want to build an impressive physique you have to devote your life to training and live in the gym. Well, that's not the case. And besides, they don't like you sleeping under the squat rack.

The truth is that three 40-minute sessions a week is all you need, provided they are sessions containing the right exercises performed with the right set and rep ranges. That's where this plan comes in. Over six months you work on every major muscle group, using exercises that give you the biggest bang for your buck and set and rep ranges that will improve strength and also make your muscle grow. And as your muscles grow you'll also notice that your body fat levels fall. So ask yourself this question: can you spare 40 minutes three times a week?

YOUR BEST BODY COUNTDOWN

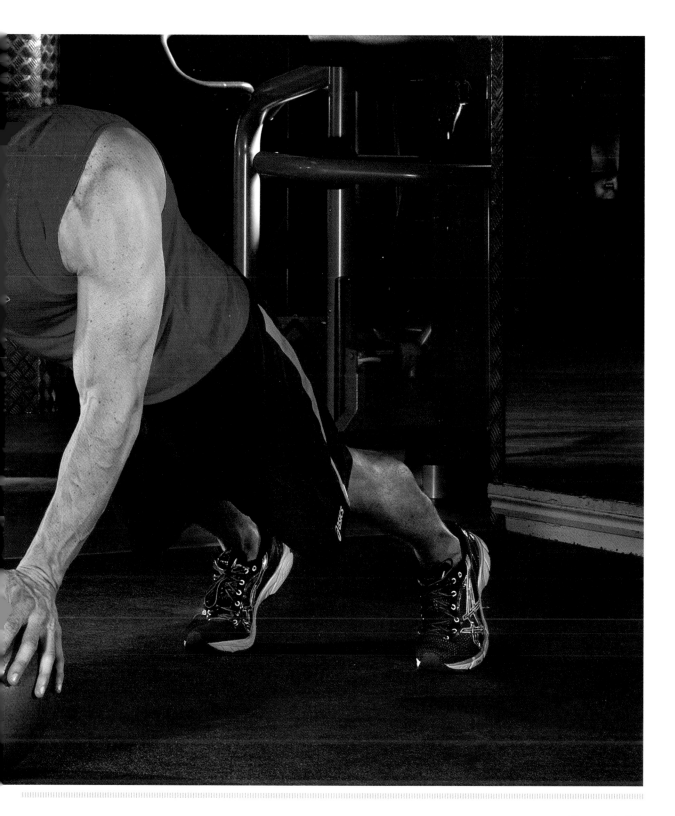

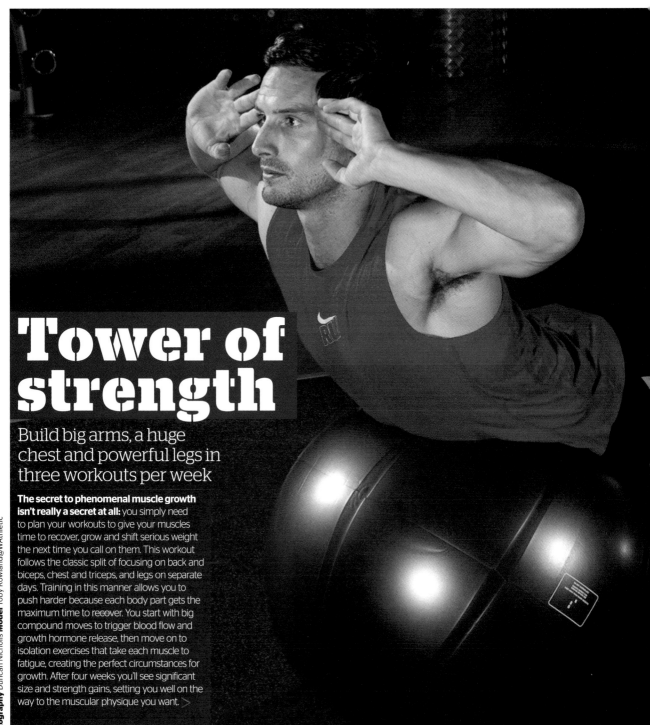

Tower of strength

Build big arms, a huge chest and powerful legs in three workouts per week

The secret to phenomenal muscle growth isn't really a secret at all: you simply need to plan your workouts to give your muscles time to recover, grow and shift serious weight the next time you call on them. This workout follows the classic split of focusing on back and biceps, chest and triceps, and legs on separate days. Training in this manner allows you to push harder because each body part gets the maximum time to recover. You start with big compound moves to trigger blood flow and growth hormone release, then move on to isolation exercises that take each muscle to fatigue, creating the perfect circumstances for growth. After four weeks you'll see significant size and strength gains, setting you well on the way to the muscular physique you want. ▷

Photography Duncan Nicholls **Model** Toby Rowland@WAthletic

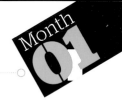

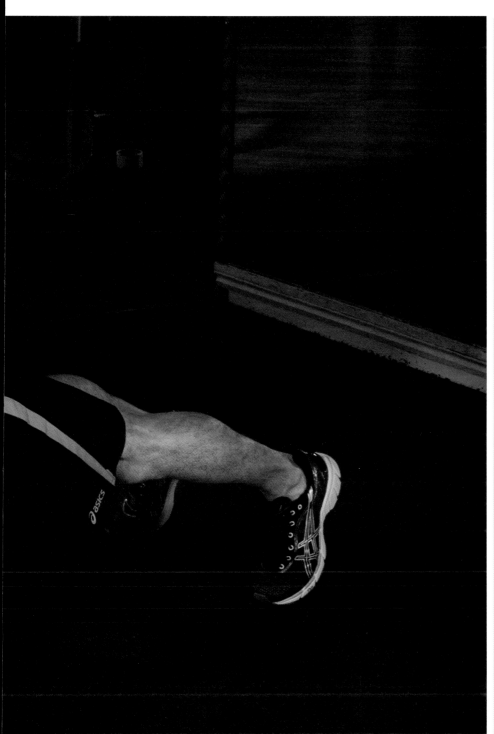

How to do it

 Timing Workouts should take about 30 minutes, including the warm-up.

 Warm-up Spend five minutes doing bodyweight moves such as press-ups, squats and lunges.

 Weight Choose a weight that allows you to complete all your reps but no more.

 Tempo Take one second to lift the weight, pause, then take three seconds to lower.

 Rest Rest for 30-45 seconds between sets and for one minute between exercises.

How you do it

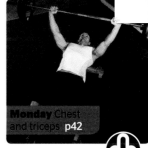
Monday Chest and triceps **p42**

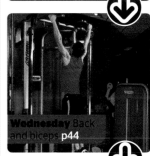
Wednesday Back and biceps **p44**

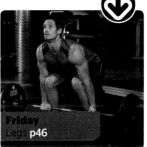
Friday Legs **p46**

Month 01

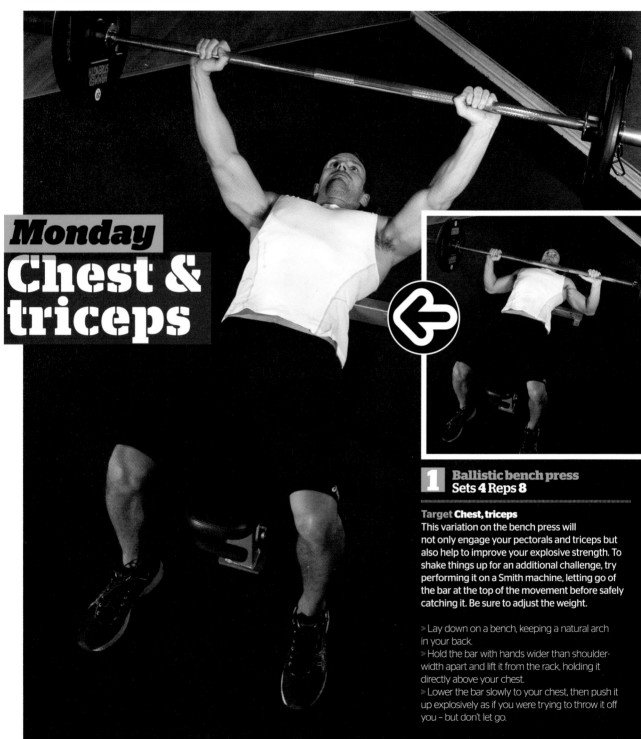

Monday
Chest & triceps

1 Ballistic bench press
Sets 4 Reps 8

Target Chest, triceps

This variation on the bench press will not only engage your pectorals and triceps but also help to improve your explosive strength. To shake things up for an additional challenge, try performing it on a Smith machine, letting go of the bar at the top of the movement before safely catching it. Be sure to adjust the weight.

> Lay down on a bench, keeping a natural arch in your back.
> Hold the bar with hands wider than shoulder-width apart and lift it from the rack, holding it directly above your chest.
> Lower the bar slowly to your chest, then push it up explosively as if you were trying to throw it off you – but don't let go.

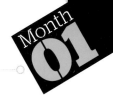

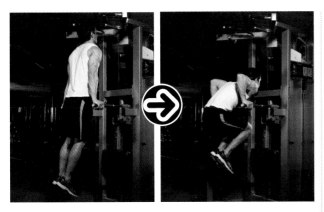

2 Fold dip
Sets 4 Reps 6-8

Target Triceps, abs
Another variation on a classic, this will target triceps and abs in a different way to challenge your body after the bench press. The targeted muscles will grow as well as strengthening your core.
> Grip the bars either side of your waist.
> Lean forward to take pressure off your shoulders and draw in your knees as you dip.

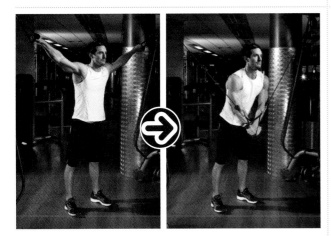

4 Cable crossover
Sets 3 Reps 12

Target Chest
This will put the pectorals under a constant state of tension, taking them a step closer to being completely fatigued.
> Stand in the centre of a cable crossover machine and hold both cables, placing some of the tension

in your arms.
> Stand with feet hip-width apart and lean forward from the hips slightly.
> Pull the cables into the middle until your hands touch, then return to the start of the move.

3 Diamond press-up
Sets 3 Reps 12

Target Chest, triceps
With your chest and triceps starting to get fatigued, switching to this alternative version of the traditional press-up is a good way to shock your body once again. Make sure you warm your wrists up first to get the most out of the move.

> Get in a press-up position and place your hands together so your two index fingers and two thumbs are touching, creating a diamond.
> Bend your elbows and lower your chest to the floor before pushing back up to the starting position.

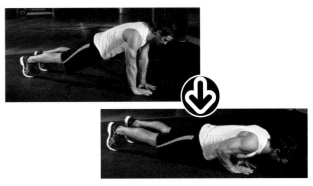

5 One arm press-down
Sets 2 Reps 10 each side

Target Triceps
Using only one arm in this classic move allows you to home in on the muscle while concentrating on form.
> Set the cable at head height and stand up with your back straight.
> Tuck your elbow into your side and pull the handle down.
> Squeeze your triceps at the bottom of the move before returning to the starting point.

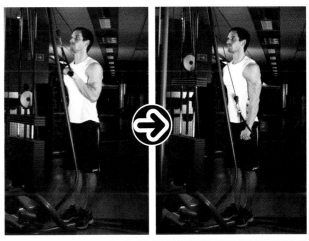

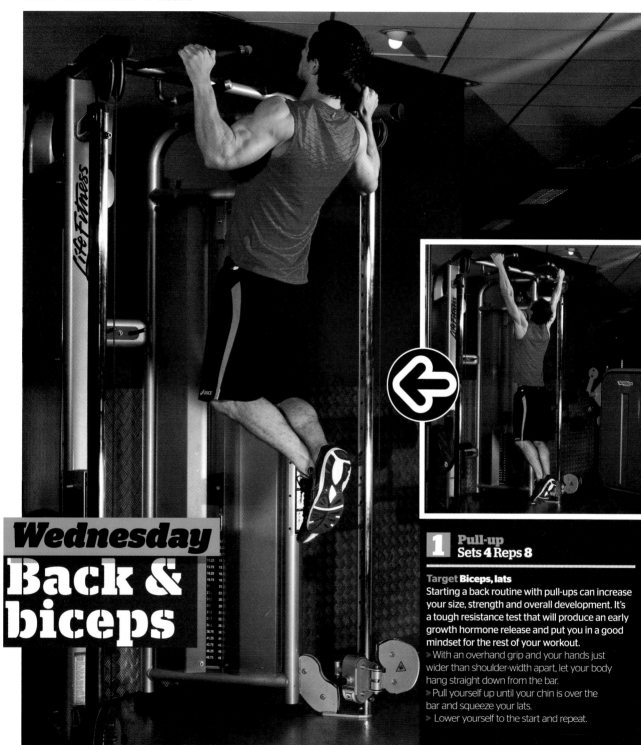

Wednesday
Back & biceps

1 | Pull-up
Sets 4 Reps 8

Target Biceps, lats

Starting a back routine with pull-ups can increase your size, strength and overall development. It's a tough resistance test that will produce an early growth hormone release and put you in a good mindset for the rest of your workout.

➤ With an overhand grip and your hands just wider than shoulder-width apart, let your body hang straight down from the bar.

➤ Pull yourself up until your chin is over the bar and squeeze your lats.

➤ Lower yourself to the start and repeat.

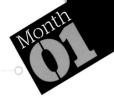

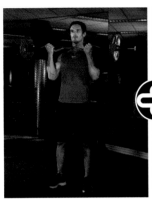
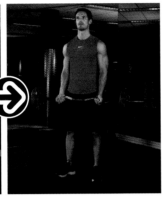

3 Dumb-bell shrug
Sets 3 Reps 12

Target Traps
The shrug is essential for building the upper back, which frequently comes under strain from other exercises.
> Grasp a dumb-bell in each hand and hold them by your sides with your palms facing your body.
> Retract your shoulder blades and maintain a natural arch in your back.
> Use your traps to lift the weights. Hold the up position for one to two seconds.

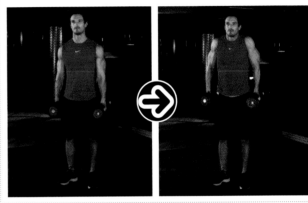

2 EZ-bar biceps curl
Sets 4 Reps 8

Target Biceps
Despite the name, using the EZ-bar isn't an easy option – it takes the strain of curling off your wrists and elbows to focus on your biceps.
> Stand with feet hip-width apart, holding an EZ-bar at hip height.
> Keeping your elbows close to your sides, squeeze your biceps to curl the bar up to shoulder level
> Lower the bar slowly back to the start position.

5 Gym ball back extension
Sets 3 Reps 10

Target Lats
Your lower back may get a good workout from deadlifts, but for a balanced physique it needs to be worked more directly. This exercise will do just that, bringing your workout to a strong finish.
> Lie face down on a gym ball with your feet shoulder-width apart.
> Slightly bend your knees for balance and then curl your chin towards the ball before extending up, bringing your elbows back.

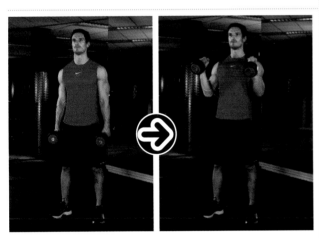

4 Hammer curl
Sets 3 Reps 10

Target Biceps, forearms
Targeting both the biceps and the forearms will aid your overall development as well as increasing your grip strength.
> Begin by tucking your elbows in to your sides and grip two dumb-bells with your palms facing in.
> Curl the weights up to your chest, maintaining the hammer grip throughout the movement.

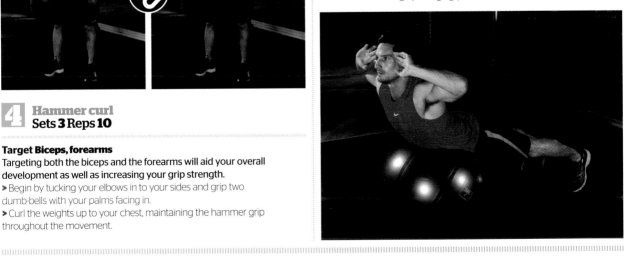

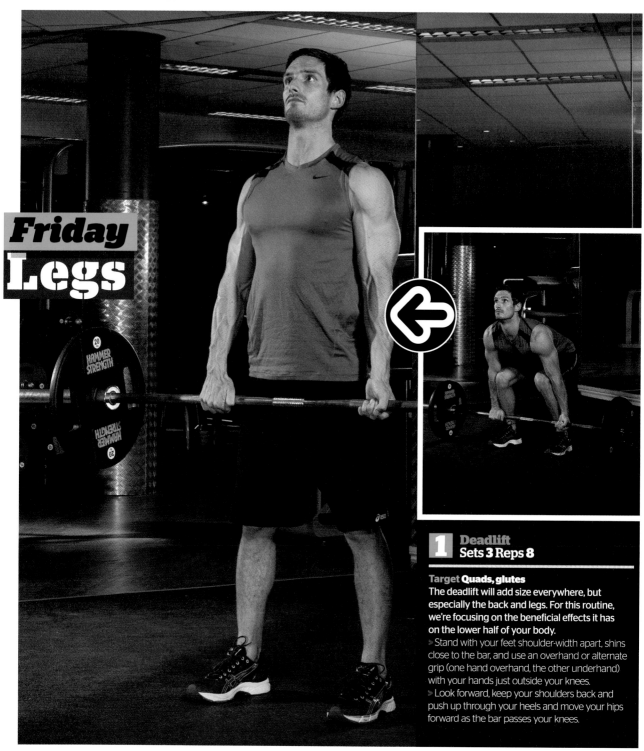

Friday
Legs

1 Deadlift
Sets 3 Reps 8

Target Quads, glutes
The deadlift will add size everywhere, but especially the back and legs. For this routine, we're focusing on the beneficial effects it has on the lower half of your body.
➤ Stand with your feet shoulder-width apart, shins close to the bar, and use an overhand or alternate grip (one hand overhand, the other underhand) with your hands just outside your knees.
➤ Look forward, keep your shoulders back and push up through your heels and move your hips forward as the bar passes your knees.

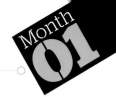

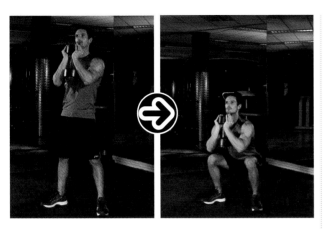

② Sumo squat
Sets **3** Reps **10**

Target Quads
While the standard squat is still a worthy part of any routine, the best way to exhaust your legs is to introduce the sumo variation after performing some deadlifts. It hits your inner quads particularly hard.

> Take a wide stance and point your toes outwards.
> Hold a dumb-bell by its end and squat down until the weight is just above your knees.
> Finish the move by pushing back up through your heels.

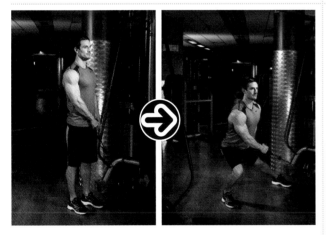

④ Cable side lunge
Sets **2** Reps **10 each side**

Target Quads, hamstrings, glutes
A complete workout for your legs, with the bonus of hitting your glutes as well. This will take the target muscles close to exhaustion.

> Stand side-on to a cable machine with a D-handle attached to the bottom clip.
> Reach across your body and grasp the handle, then take a big step to the side, bending your leading leg as it lands.
> Reverse the move back to the start and repeat on both sides.

③ Step-up
Sets **2** Reps **10 each side**

Target: Quads, glutes
A top move for functional strength – we all use stairs every day – and it hits the typically under-trained glutes as well as the quads.

> Look forward and keep your back upright.
> Hold dumb-bells by your side and step up with one leg.
> Step down with your trailing leg and repeat, then switch legs.

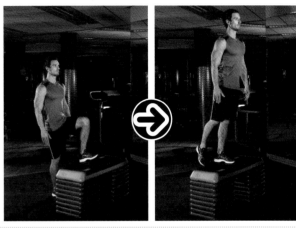

⑤ Calf raise
Sets **2** Reps **10 each side**

Target Calves
Your legs should be fully fatigued by now, so it's time to shift to your calves.
> Place the ball of your foot on the edge of a step. Let your non-working foot hang free. Hold a dumb-bell by your side and hold a wall for balance if needed.
> Push up until your heel is as high as it can go, holding the tension at the top.
> Lower slowly to the start, repeat as before and then switch legs.

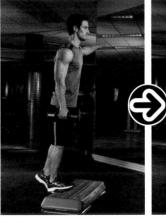
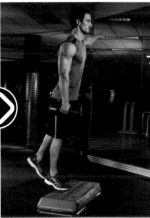

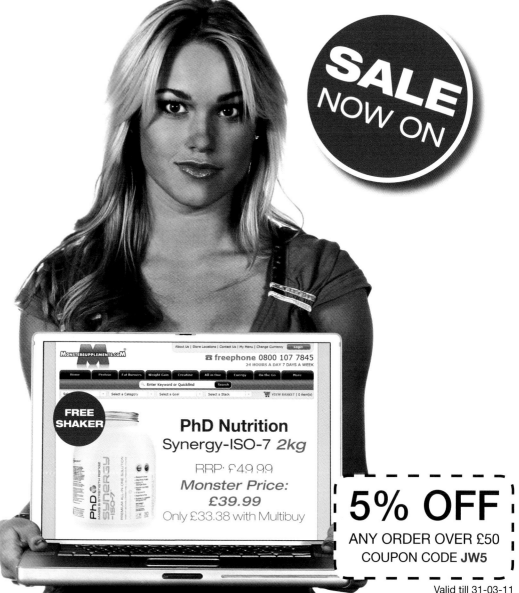
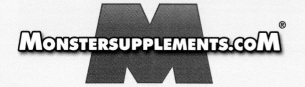

Month 02

Push yourself

Building muscles is simple: push them to the limit, then let them recover before pushing them again

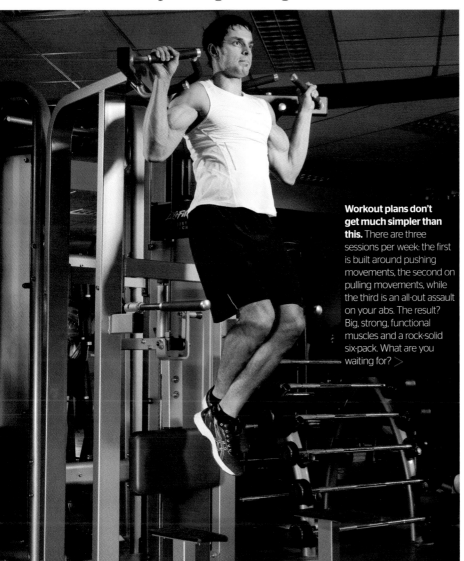

Workout plans don't get much simpler than this. There are three sessions per week: the first is built around pushing movements, the second on pulling movements, while the third is an all-out assault on your abs. The result? Big, strong, functional muscles and a rock-solid six-pack. What are you waiting for? >

Photography Duncan Nicholls Model Richard Scrivener@WAthletic

How to do it

 Timing Workouts should take about 30 minutes, including the warm-up.

 Warm-up Spend five minutes doing bodyweight moves such as press-ups, squats and lunges.

 Weight Choose a weight that allows you to complete all your reps but no more.

 Tempo Take one second to lift the weight, pause, then take three seconds to lower.

 Rest Rest for 30-45 seconds between sets and for one minute between exercises.

How you do it

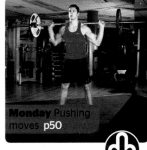
Monday Pushing moves **p50**

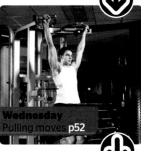
Wednesday Pulling moves **p52**

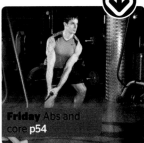
Friday Abs and core **p54**

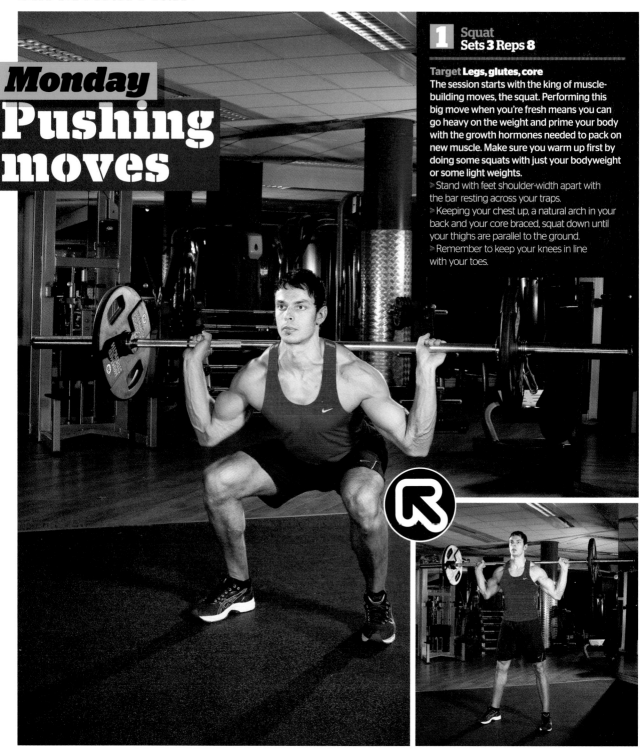

Monday
Pushing moves

1 Squat
Sets 3 Reps 8

Target Legs, glutes, core

The session starts with the king of muscle-building moves, the squat. Performing this big move when you're fresh means you can go heavy on the weight and prime your body with the growth hormones needed to pack on new muscle. Make sure you warm up first by doing some squats with just your bodyweight or some light weights.

≫ Stand with feet shoulder-width apart with the bar resting across your traps.

≫ Keeping your chest up, a natural arch in your back and your core braced, squat down until your thighs are parallel to the ground.

≫ Remember to keep your knees in line with your toes.

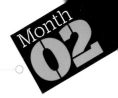

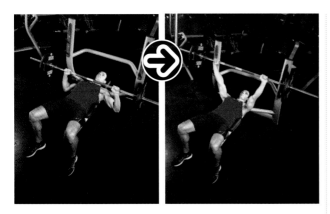

2 Bench press
Sets 3 Reps 8

Target Chest, shoulders, triceps
The best move for sculpting a big chest. Doing two big moves back to back will produce lots of muscle-building hormones.
> Lie flat on a bench with your feet planted on the floor.
> Hold the bar with a shoulder-width overhand grip.
> Keeping your glutes and upper back against the bench, slowly lower the bar to your chest before pushing back up.
> Don't lock out your arms.

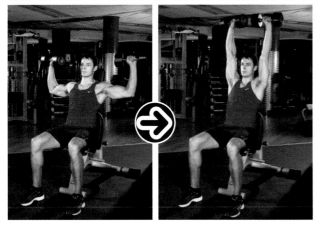

4 Seated dumb-bell press
Sets 3 Reps 10

Target Shoulders, triceps
Stay seated for a more stable base that allows you to lift more weight.
> Sit on a bench with your feet flat on the floor.

> Hold a dumb-bell in each hand at shoulder height.
> Keeping your core braced, press the weights above your head, then slowly return.

3 Step-up jump
Sets 3 Reps 12

Target Legs, glutes, core
Performing these explosive jumps will work your fast-twitch muscles fibres, which respond well to growth stimulus, while also firing up your heart rate to help mobilise fat stores for burning.

> Stand in front of a box or bench that's between ankle and knee height.
> Squat slightly then power up explosively to land with both feet on the box.
> Step back down and repeat.

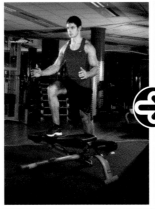
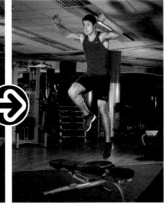

5 Diamond press-up
Sets 3 Reps To failure

Target Chest, triceps, core
The final move of the session again focuses on the major upper-body muscles. Because this is the last exercise, keep performing reps in each set until you can't do any more with good form.
> Start in a press-up position, but with thumbs and index fingers forming a diamond.
> Slowly lower your chest.
> When you're about fist-distance from the ground, press back up.

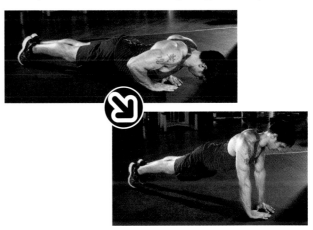

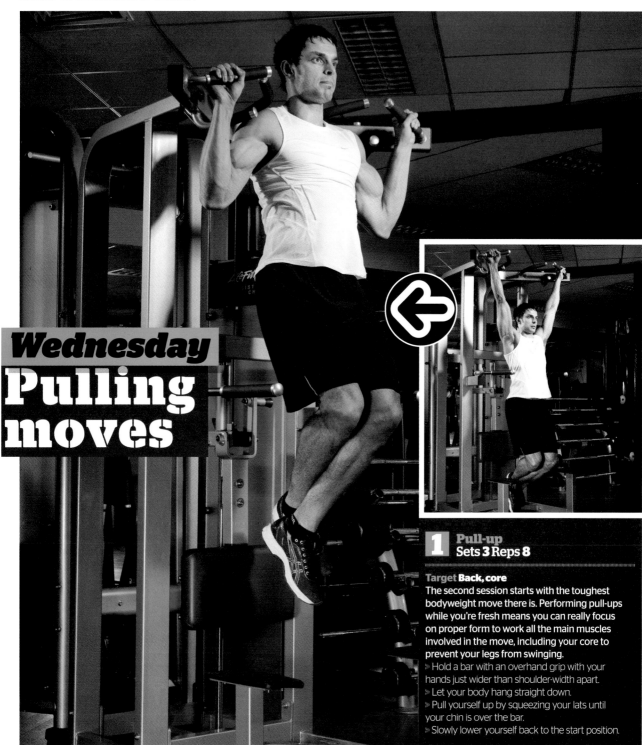

Wednesday
Pulling moves

1 Pull-up
Sets 3 Reps 8

Target Back, core

The second session starts with the toughest bodyweight move there is. Performing pull-ups while you're fresh means you can really focus on proper form to work all the main muscles involved in the move, including your core to prevent your legs from swinging.

➤ Hold a bar with an overhand grip with your hands just wider than shoulder-width apart.
➤ Let your body hang straight down.
➤ Pull yourself up by squeezing your lats until your chin is over the bar.
➤ Slowly lower yourself back to the start position.

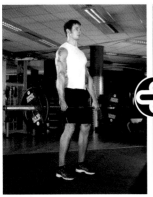 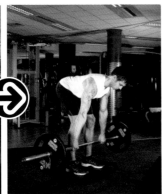

3 One-arm cable row
Sets 3 Reps 12

Target Traps, lats, rhomboids, biceps
Cable rows target the powerful muscles in your upper back and also tax your biceps. The cable maintains resistance throughout the move. Don't use momentum and perform each rep slowly.
> Stand at a cable machine with the attachment at the bottom.
> With a bend in your knees, your core braced and a natural arch in your back, hold the handle with a neutral (palms together) grip.
> Pull the handle to your sternum, squeezing your shoulder blades together.

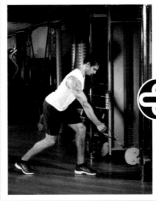 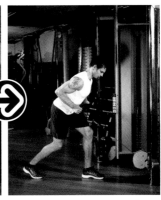

2 Romanian deadlift
Sets 3 Reps 8

Target Lower back, hamstrings
This tough move is the best way to pack on muscle on the back of your thighs. Make sure your form is perfect to avoid unnecessary strain on your lower back.
> Stand with feet shoulder-width apart, holding a bar with an overhand grip slightly wider than your hips.
> With your shoulders back and core braced, lean forward from the hips, not the waist.
> Lower the bar slowly down your shins until you feel the stretch in your hamstrings.

5 Biceps curl
Sets 3 Reps 12

Target Biceps
The session ends by blitzing your biceps and forearms.
> Stand with a dumb-bell in each hand, with palms facing each other.
> Brace your core and keep your elbows tucked in to your sides.
> Curl the weights up, rotating your wrists until they're at shoulder height.
> Return slowly to the start – don't rock back and forth for momentum.

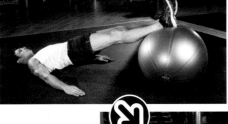 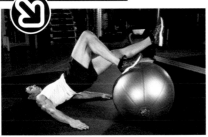

4 Single-leg gym ball hamstring curl
Sets 3 Reps 8

Target Hamstrings, core
This works your core and legs to improve stability.
> Lie with one foot on a gym ball and your body straight.
> Raise your hips and drag the ball back with your heel. Pause, then slowly return to the start.

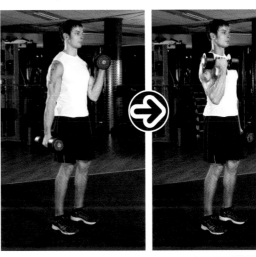

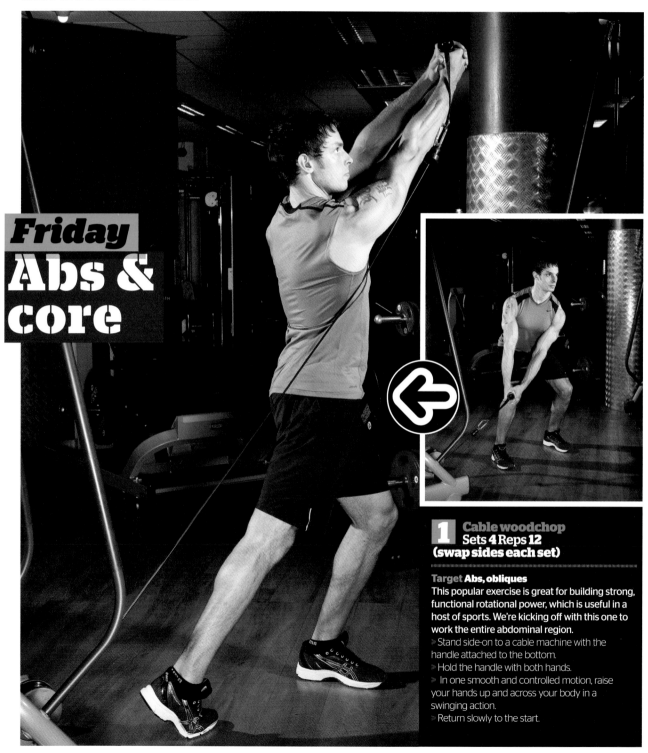

Friday
Abs & core

1 Cable woodchop
Sets 4 Reps 12
(swap sides each set)

Target Abs, obliques

This popular exercise is great for building strong, functional rotational power, which is useful in a host of sports. We're kicking off with this one to work the entire abdominal region.

> Stand side-on to a cable machine with the handle attached to the bottom.

> Hold the handle with both hands.

> In one smooth and controlled motion, raise your hands up and across your body in a swinging action.

> Return slowly to the start.

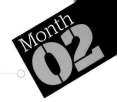

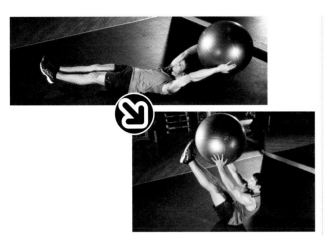

2 Gym ball passing jackknife
Sets 3 Reps 12

Target Abs

Moving the ball back and forth from your hands to your feet engages the entire core region in two ways: crunching up and drawing your legs towards your chest works your top, middle and lower abs, while your deeper stability muscles must hold your torso stable throughout every rep.

> Hold a gym ball behind your head with your arms straight.
> Crunch up and raise your feet so you can place the ball between them.
> Extend your legs back out and hold for a second before returning the ball to your hands and repeating.

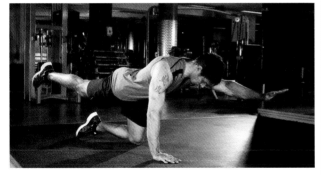

4 Two-point box
Sets 3 Reps 12

Target Abs

The penultimate move in the workout requires a strong core, and also demands a great deal of co-ordination.

> Kneel on the floor and place your hands directly underneath your shoulders.
> Draw the opposing knee and elbow together so they touch under your stomach, then extend your leg and arm away from your torso.
> Return back to the start position and repeat with opposite limbs.

3 Seated Russian twist
Sets 4 Reps 12

Target Abs, obliques

This is another rotational move to test your obliques and those deeper core muscles that stabilise your body and allow you to transfer power between your upper and lower body.

> Sit on the floor with your torso held at an angle of 45° to the floor and your knees bent at 90°.
> Hold a dumb-bell with both hands and twist one way.
> With torso and knees at the same angle, twist the other way.
> Use your abs to control the motion, rather than swinging back and forth.

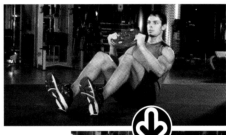

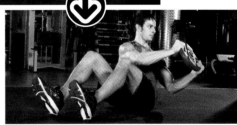

5 Gym ball plank
Sets 4 Time 30-45sec

Target Abs

The instability of the gym ball makes this move far harder – and therefore far better for building solid abs – than a normal plank.

> Start in a plank position with your elbows on a gym ball.
> Brace your core and keep your body in a straight line.
> Don't let your hips sag.

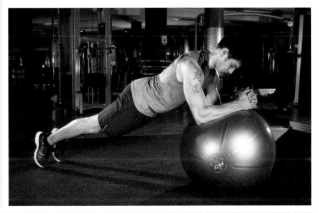

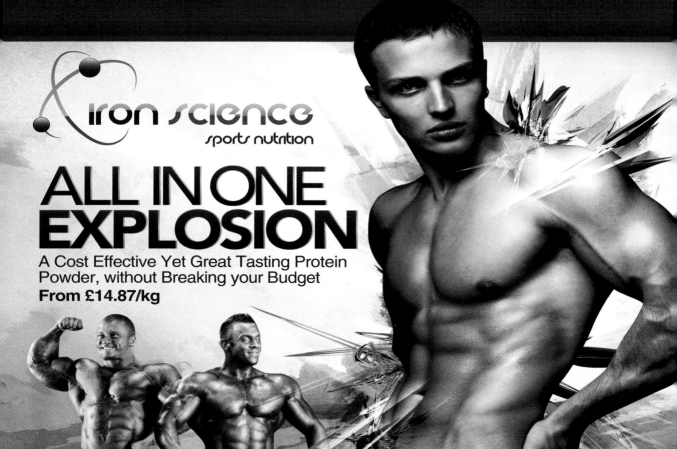
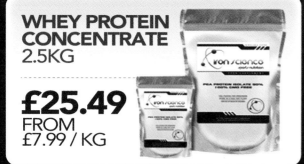

Whole-body muscle plan

Build muscle all over your body with this three-part plan

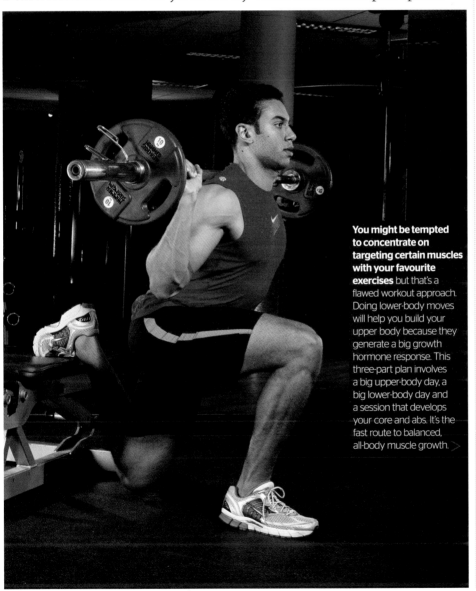

You might be tempted to concentrate on targeting certain muscles with your favourite exercises but that's a flawed workout approach. Doing lower-body moves will help you build your upper body because they generate a big growth hormone response. This three-part plan involves a big upper-body day, a big lower-body day and a session that develops your core and abs. It's the fast route to balanced, all-body muscle growth.

Photography Duncan Nicholls Model Mark Hughes@WAthletic

How to do it

 Timing Each muscle-building session should take approximately 40 minutes, including the warm-up.

 Warm-up Spend five minutes doing bodyweight moves such as squats and press-ups. Before each big move, do a warm-up set with a very light weight.

 Weight Choose a weight that allows you to complete all your reps but no more.

Tempo Take one second to lift the weight, pause, then take three seconds to lower.

Rest Rest for one minute between sets and two minutes between exercises.

How you do it

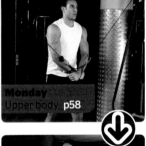
Monday Upper body p58

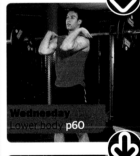
Wednesday Lower body p60

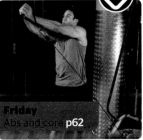
Friday Abs and core p62

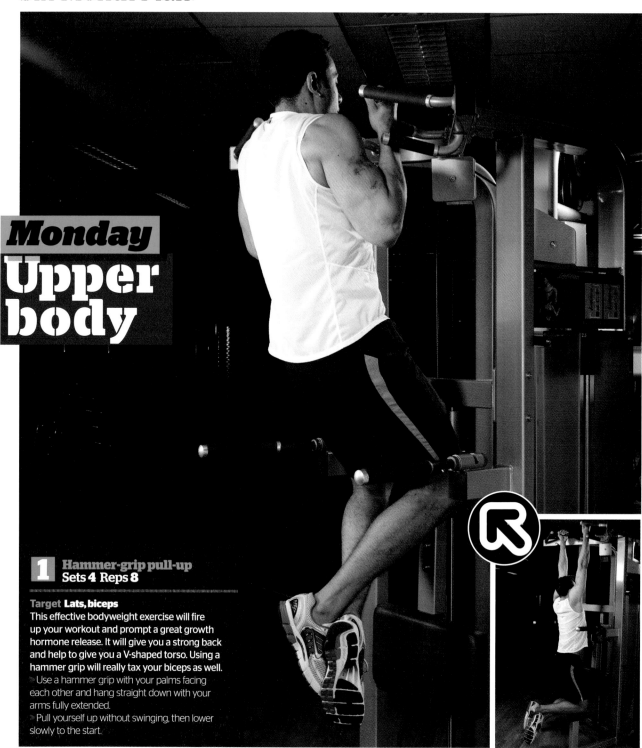

Monday
Upper body

1 **Hammer-grip pull-up**
Sets 4 Reps 8

Target Lats, biceps
This effective bodyweight exercise will fire
up your workout and prompt a great growth
hormone release. It will give you a strong back
and help to give you a V-shaped torso. Using a
hammer grip will really tax your biceps as well.
≫ Use a hammer grip with your palms facing
each other and hang straight down with your
arms fully extended.
≫ Pull yourself up without swinging, then lower
slowly to the start.

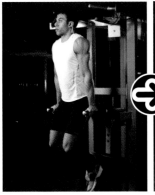
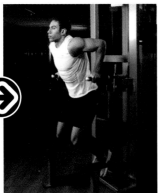

2 Dip
Sets 4 Reps 6-8

Target Triceps, chest
Follow the hammer-grip pull-up with another classic bodyweight move. It's a great exercise to do here because it's tough but taxes different muscles to the first move. It'll make your triceps bigger and stronger, and will also work your chest.

> Grip the dip bars with your arms straight and your body upright.
> Bend at the elbows to lower your body, making sure your elbows point backwards.
> Lower as far as is comfortable, then push back to the start.

3 Shoulder press
Sets 3 Reps 10

Target Shoulders
The final upper body part that's yet to be worked, your shoulders, is targeted by this big compound move. By using a barbell you can lift heavy weights, which will lead to big muscle and strength improvements.

> Hold the bar just wider than shoulder-width apart and rest it on the top of your chest.
> Press the bar directly overhead, then lower to the start.

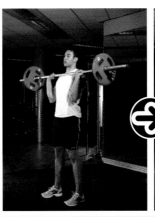
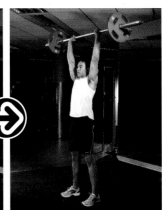

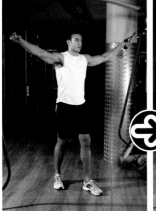
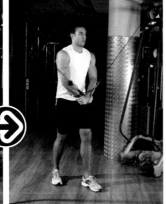

4 Cable crossover
Sets 3 Reps 10

Target Chest
You've done all the big compound moves so now it's time to focus in on key muscles. This move isolates your chest and the cable keeps the tension constant throughout the move.

> Stand in the middle of a cable crossover machine with your arms out holding the cables so that there is some tension in them.
> Use a split stance with your weight over your front foot.
> Draw the cables into the middle until your hands touch.

5 Barbell biceps curl
Sets 3 Reps 10

Target Biceps
The final move of the workout lets you fully fatigue your biceps after you've worked them in the hammer-grip pull-up. They've had a good chance to recover from that move, so you can still lift a heavy weight.

> Hold the barbell by your thighs, then curl it up to your chest
> Make sure you don't rock back because that would mean you're using momentum to help you lift the weight.

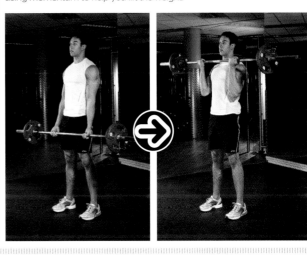

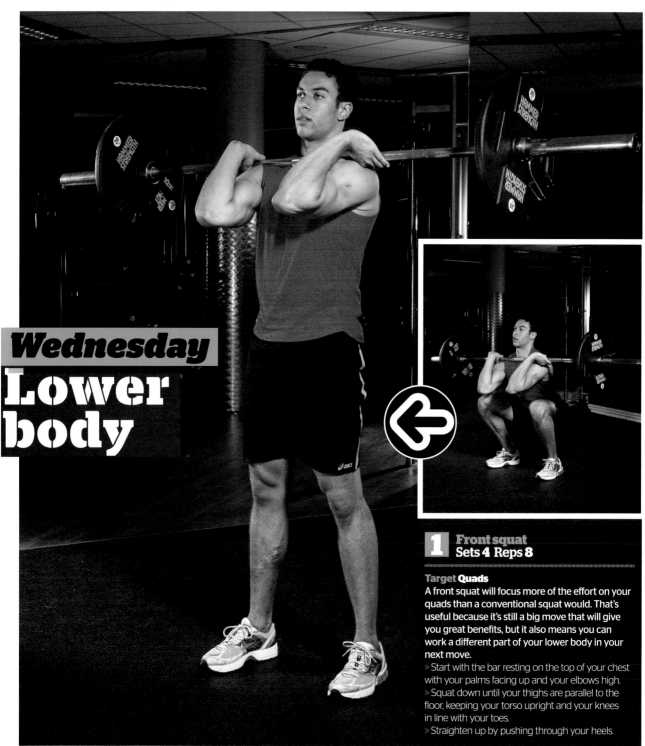

Wednesday
Lower body

1 Front squat
Sets 4 Reps 8

Target Quads

A front squat will focus more of the effort on your quads than a conventional squat would. That's useful because it's still a big move that will give you great benefits, but it also means you can work a different part of your lower body in your next move.

➤ Start with the bar resting on the top of your chest with your palms facing up and your elbows high.
➤ Squat down until your thighs are parallel to the floor, keeping your torso upright and your knees in line with your toes.
➤ Straighten up by pushing through your heels.

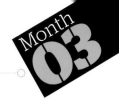

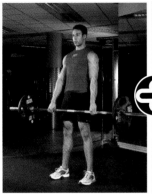
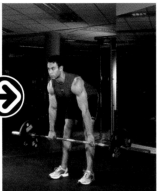

2 Romanian deadlift
Sets **4** Reps **8**

Target Hamstrings, glutes
The first exercise in this workout targeted the front of your thighs. This one focuses on the back as well as recruiting the glutes. Both those muscles are often under-trained, so this is important for balanced growth.

> Stand with your knees slightly bent and rest the barbell on your thighs.
> Bend from the hips, rather than the waist, to send the bar down the front of your legs until you feel a strong stretch in your hamstrings.

3 Bulgarian split squat
Sets **2** Reps **6-8 each side**

Target Quads, glutes
This exercise requires a lot of concentration to stay balanced so it works your stabilising muscles. You're also going back to working your quads while your hamstrings recover.

> Stand with one foot on a bench and your other foot planted one stride in front of the bench.
> Rest the barbell on your back with your torso upright.
> Bend your knees to lower into the squat, keeping your torso upright and your front knee in line with your toes.

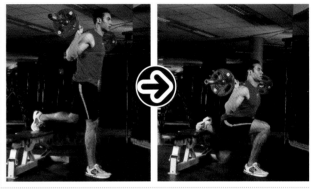

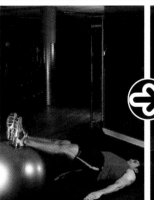
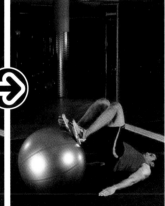

4 Gym ball hamstring curl
Sets **3** Reps **10**

Target Hamstrings
By now your quads will be fatigued, so this move is all about hamstring and glute strength and stability. It takes effort to control the movement of the ball as you drag it towards your backside.

> Lie on your back with your calves resting on the ball.
> Lift your hips and drag the ball in towards your backside until your body is straight from knees to shoulders.

5 One-leg glute bridge
Sets **3** Reps **10**

Target Glutes
The final move in the workout targets your glutes. Strong glutes will make you a better runner and are also vital for performing big, demanding exercises, such as deadlifts.

> Lie on the floor with one knee bent and the other leg straight and off the floor.
> Raise your backside off the ground so your body is straight from knees to shoulders.

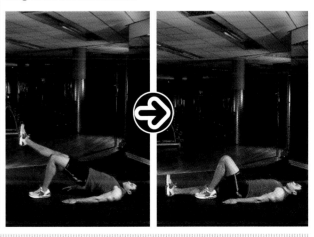

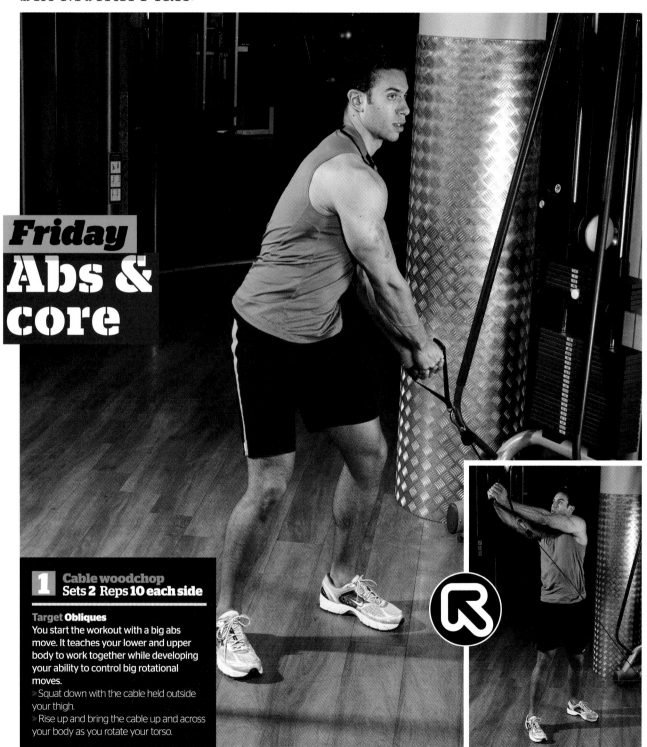

Friday
Abs & core

1 Cable woodchop
Sets 2 Reps 10 each side

Target Obliques

You start the workout with a big abs move. It teaches your lower and upper body to work together while developing your ability to control big rotational moves.

≫ Squat down with the cable held outside your thigh.

≫ Rise up and bring the cable up and across your body as you rotate your torso.

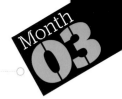

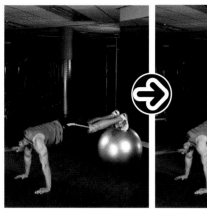
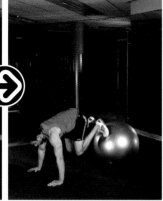

2 Gym ball jackknife
Sets 3 Reps 10

Target Abs
While your abs are still relatively fresh you can do this challenging move. It works your upper, middle and lower abs, as well as recruiting your obliques, which work to make sure

you don't fall off the ball.
> Begin in a press-up position with your feet resting on the gym ball.
> Bend your knees to draw the ball towards you, without raising your backside.

3 Twisting knee raise
Sets 3 Reps 5 each side

Target Lower abs
The lower abs are the hardest part of your midsection to hit. This move will home in on that area. Once it becomes easy, make it harder either by doing it with a medicine ball between your legs.
> Take an overhand grip and hang straight down from the bar.
> Keeping your upper body still, bend your knees, raise your legs and twist to one side.

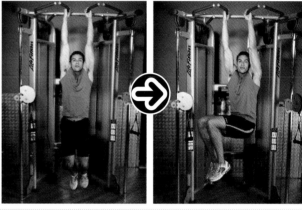

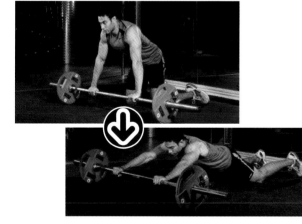

4 Barbell rollout
Sets 3 Reps 10

Target Abs, core
This is a difficult but highly effective exercise. It puts your upper body in a very unstable position so your abs, core and lower back all have to work to keep your spine stable.
> Start on your knees with your core braced, your spine in a neutral position and the barbell directly below your shoulders.
> Keeping your core braced, roll the bar forwards as far as you can without curving your spine.

5 Side plank
Sets 2 Time 30-45 seconds

Target Obliques, core
The session ends with a static hold. This type of exercise is great for your core and for developing the deep-lying muscles that support your spine. By doing this exercise you'll become better prepared for doing big lifts.
> Position yourself so your elbow is directly beneath your shoulder and your body is straight from head to heels.
> Hold that position for the required time or until your hips sag.

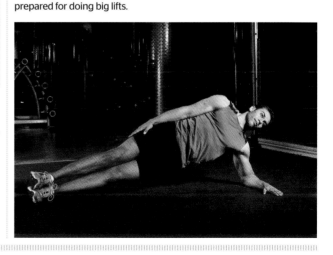

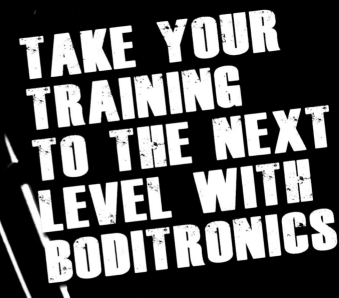
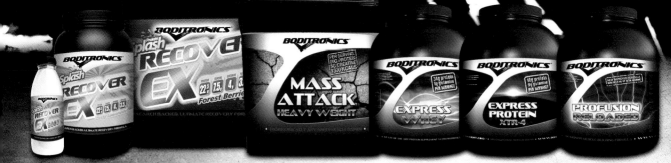

Solid build

Work on each part of your body separately to pack on muscle all over

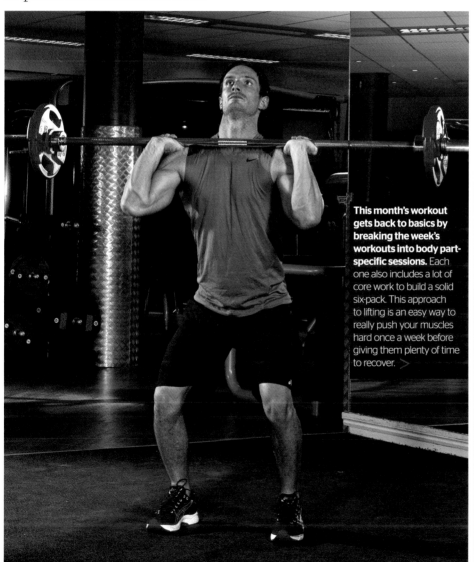

This month's workout gets back to basics by breaking the week's workouts into body part-specific sessions. Each one also includes a lot of core work to build a solid six-pack. This approach to lifting is an easy way to really push your muscles hard once a week before giving them plenty of time to recover. ▷

How to do it

 Timing Workouts should take about 30 minutes, including the warm-up.

 Warm-up Spend five minutes doing bodyweight moves such as press-ups, squats and lunges.

 Weight Choose a weight that allows you to complete all your reps but no more.

 Tempo Take one second to lift the weight, pause, then take three seconds to lower.

 Rest Rest for 30-45 seconds between sets and for one minute between exercises.

How you do it

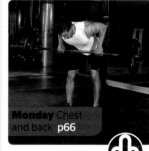

Monday Chest and back **p66**

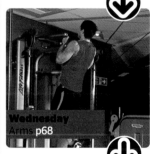

Wednesday Arms **p68**

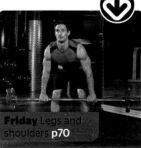

Friday Legs and shoulders **p70**

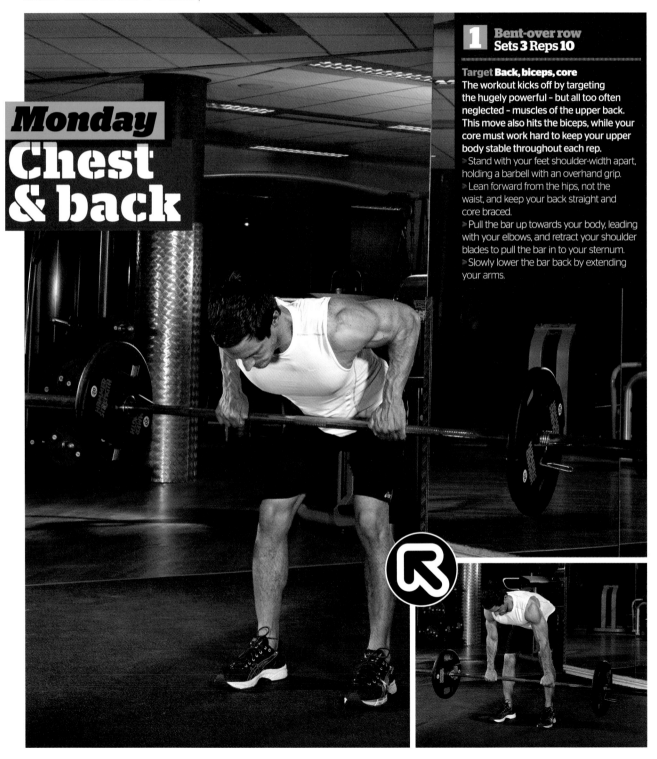

Monday
Chest & back

1 Bent-over row
Sets 3 Reps 10

Target Back, biceps, core

The workout kicks off by targeting the hugely powerful – but all too often neglected – muscles of the upper back. This move also hits the biceps, while your core must work hard to keep your upper body stable throughout each rep.

➤ Stand with your feet shoulder-width apart, holding a barbell with an overhand grip.
➤ Lean forward from the hips, not the waist, and keep your back straight and core braced.
➤ Pull the bar up towards your body, leading with your elbows, and retract your shoulder blades to pull the bar in to your sternum.
➤ Slowly lower the bar back by extending your arms.

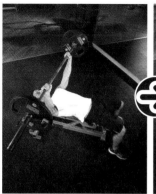
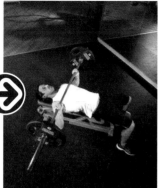

3 Lat pull-down
Sets 3 Reps 10

Target Back, biceps
Your lats are hugely powerful muscles that help create a strong V-shaped torso. This move works the lats through their full range of motion, so keep each rep slow and controlled to maximise results.

> Sit at the machine with your feet flat on the floor.
> With a wide, overhand grip, slowly pull the bar down until it is just under your chin.
> Pause briefly, then slowly return it to the top.

2 Bench press
Sets 3 Reps 10

Target Chest, triceps
The king of chest moves is next. The bench press hits all the chest muscles, as well as the triceps and front of the shoulders. Ensure you lower the bar to your chest slowly so that your muscles do all the work.

> Lie flat on a bench with your feet underneath your knees.
> With a shoulder-width, overhand grip, slowly lower the bar.
> Pause briefly before pressing back up, but don't lock out your elbows.

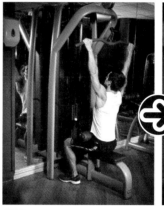
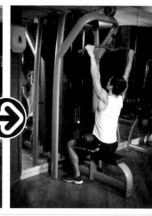

5 Good morning
Sets 3 Reps 10

Target Lower back, hamstrings, core
The final move of the session hits the muscles of the lower back, a region that, if strong, can help you lift heavier in almost every other move. The added bonus is that this exercise also hits your core and hamstrings.

> Stand with feet shoulder-width apart resting a light barbell across the top of your shoulders, not your neck.
> Keeping your lower body stable and core braced, bend forward from the hips.
> Lower your torso until you can feel a stretch in your hamstrings, then return slowly to the start.

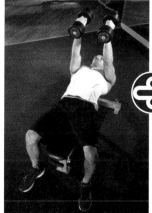
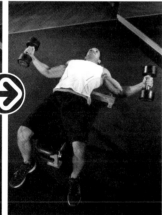

4 Dumb-bell flye
Sets 4 Reps 8

Target Chest, shoulders
This exercise focuses on your chest and the important shoulder muscles. It's vital to maintain good form throughout to avoid injury, so don't start too heavy.

> Lie on a bench holding dumb-bells above your chest.
> Slowly lower your hands out to the side, maintaining a slight bend in your elbows.
> Pause and return to the top.

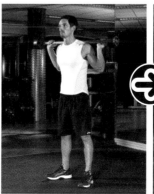
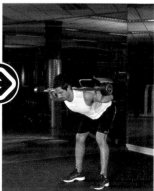

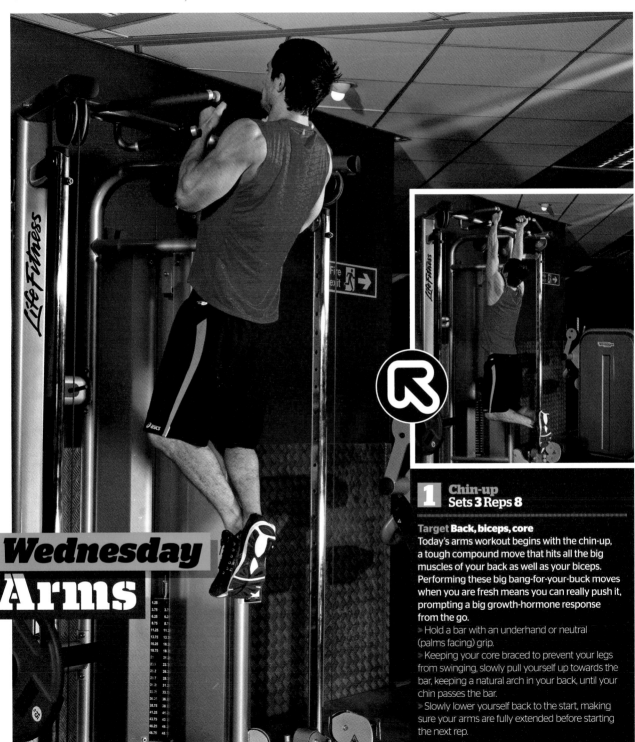

Wednesday
Arms

1 Chin-up
Sets 3 Reps 8

Target Back, biceps, core

Today's arms workout begins with the chin-up, a tough compound move that hits all the big muscles of your back as well as your biceps. Performing these big bang-for-your-buck moves when you are fresh means you can really push it, prompting a big growth-hormone response from the go.

➤ Hold a bar with an underhand or neutral (palms facing) grip.

➤ Keeping your core braced to prevent your legs from swinging, slowly pull yourself up towards the bar, keeping a natural arch in your back, until your chin passes the bar.

➤ Slowly lower yourself back to the start, making sure your arms are fully extended before starting the next rep.

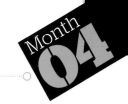

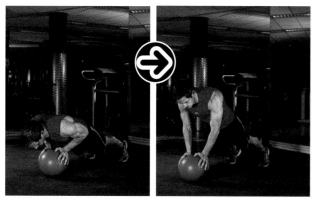

2 Medicine ball press-up
Sets 3 Reps 12

Target Chest, triceps, core
Now it's time to hit the opposite muscle groups. Using a medicine ball introduces an element of instability, forcing your core and the smaller stabilising muscles in the chest and shoulders to work harder.

> Start in a press-up position with hands on a medicine ball.
> Keeping your core braced so your body is in a straight line, slowly lower your chest until it touches the ball.
> Pause briefly, then press back up powerfully.

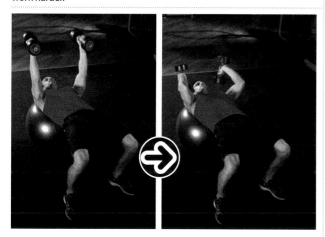

4 Gym ball lying triceps extension
Sets 3 Reps 12

Target Triceps
After three tough exercises this triceps-specific move will add size by isolating the biggest muscle of your upper arm. Remember to keep your core braced throughout to maintain balance on the ball.

> Lie with your upper back on a gym ball, holding dumb-bells directly above your chest.
> With elbows pointing to the ceiling, slowly lower the weights down to the side of your head.
> Slowly return to the start.

3 Seated dumb-bell curl
Sets 4 Reps 8

Target Biceps
After hitting the chest and triceps it's now time to tax the biceps again. Performing curls seated means you can isolate the biceps and maintain strict form: it's far harder to use momentum to 'swing' the weight up when seated than when standing up.

> Sit on a bench and hold a dumb-bell in each hand.
> Keeping your elbows tight to your body, slowly lift and twist both hands up until the weight is at shoulder height.
> Lower slowly until your arms are fully extended, then repeat.

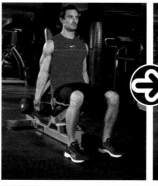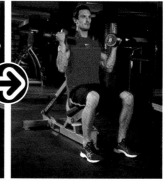

5 EZ-bar preacher curl
Sets 4 Reps 8

Target Biceps
This move will blitz your biceps and break down muscle fibres so that they grow back stronger.
> Sit at a preacher bench and hold an EZ-bar with an underhand grip.
> With your torso against the bench, slowly curl the bar up to your face.
> At the top, squeeze your biceps muscles then slowly lower the bar.

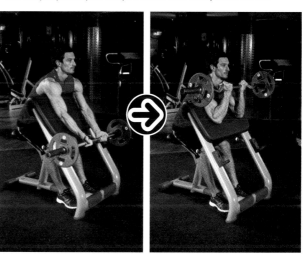

Friday
Legs & shoulders

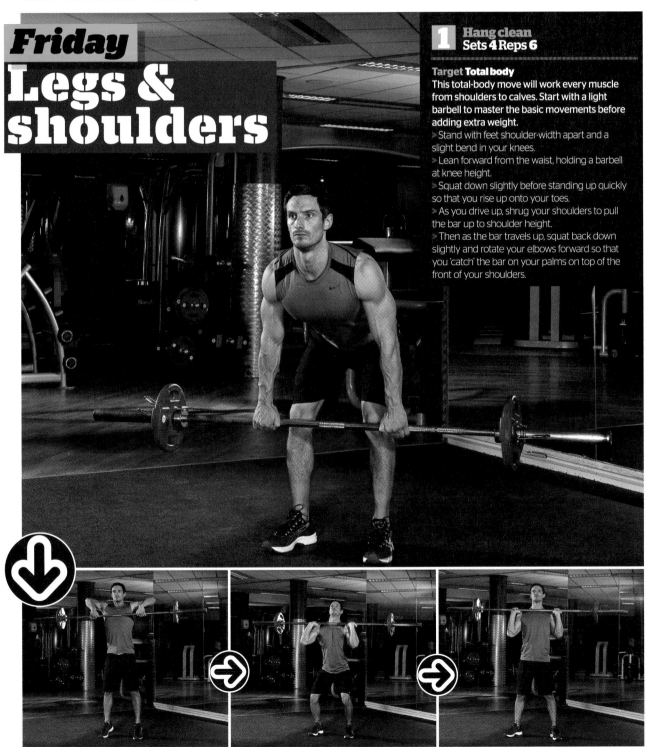

1 Hang clean
Sets 4 Reps 6

Target Total body

This total-body move will work every muscle from shoulders to calves. Start with a light barbell to master the basic movements before adding extra weight.

▸ Stand with feet shoulder-width apart and a slight bend in your knees.

▸ Lean forward from the waist, holding a barbell at knee height.

▸ Squat down slightly before standing up quickly so that you rise up onto your toes.

▸ As you drive up, shrug your shoulders to pull the bar up to shoulder height.

▸ Then as the bar travels up, squat back down slightly and rotate your elbows forward so that you 'catch' the bar on your palms on top of the front of your shoulders.

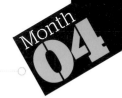

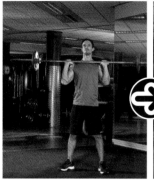
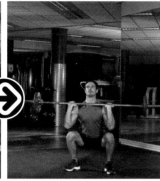

2 Front squat
Sets **4** Reps **8**

Target Quads, glutes, hamstrings, core
Resting the bar across the front of your shoulders, rather than the back of shoulders and traps, will make your quads work harder.
➤ Stand with your feet shoulder-width apart with a barbell resting on the front of your shoulders.
➤ Keeping a natural arch in your back, your core braced and your knees in line with your toes, slowly squat down until your thighs are parallel to the floor.
➤ Pause briefly before pressing through your heels to return to the start.

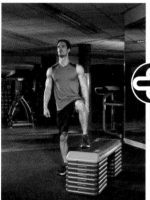
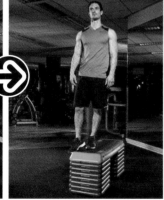

4 Side step-up
Sets **4** Reps **12**

Target Quads, glutes, hamstrings
Side step-ups work the smaller thigh muscles used in sudden lateral movements, making this a great move for improving mobility during sport.
➤ Stand side-on to a box that is about knee height.
➤ Step up on the box with one foot. Drive your body up but don't place your free foot on the box.
➤ Return to the start.
➤ Alternate legs with each set.

3 Cable reverse flye
Sets **4** Reps **8**

Target Shoulders, upper back
This move really hits your rear delts (the rear shoulder muscles), which are often ignored with standard moves.
➤ Stand between two cable weight stacks with D-handles attached at the top.
➤ Cross your arms in front of your chest, so your left hand holds the right-side cable and vice versa.
➤ Retract your shoulder blades to move your arms back and off your chest.
➤ Return to the start and repeat.

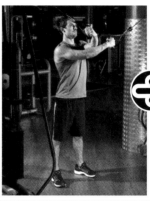
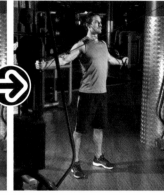

5 Alternating shoulder raise
Sets **3** Reps **10**

Target Shoulders
This final move places a lot of strain on your shoulders so always start with a light weight.
➤ Stand with feet hip-width apart holding a light dumb-bell in each hand.
➤ Keeping your core braced, raise one arm out in front and the other out to the side to shoulder height.
➤ Slowly return to the start.
➤ Alternate each arm between front and lateral raises.

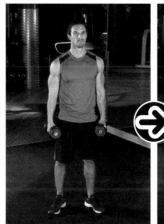
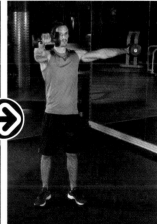

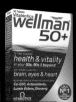
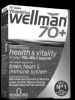
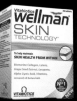
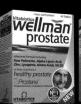

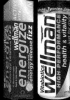

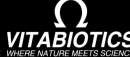

Month **05**

Power base

Build a strong core and you'll be able to lift heavier in every major move

How to do it

Timing Workouts should take about 30 minutes, including the warm-up.

Warm-up Spend five minutes doing bodyweight moves such as press-ups, squats and lunges.

Weight Choose a weight that allows you to complete all your reps but no more.

Tempo Take one second to lift the weight, pause, then take three seconds to lower.

Rest Rest for 30-45 seconds between sets and for one minute between exercises.

A house without solid foundations wouldn't last long, and the same is true of muscles. This month's workout is all about reinforcing your foundations. A strong, stable core means you will be able to lift heavier weights – especially in standing moves such as deadlifts and squats – with little risk of injury.

The three weekly workouts are split into chest and back, legs, and arms and shoulders. There is no direct abs work, but that's because your entire core region must work hard throughout most of the moves either to keep your upper body stable or because it's involved in transferring power from your lower body. ▶

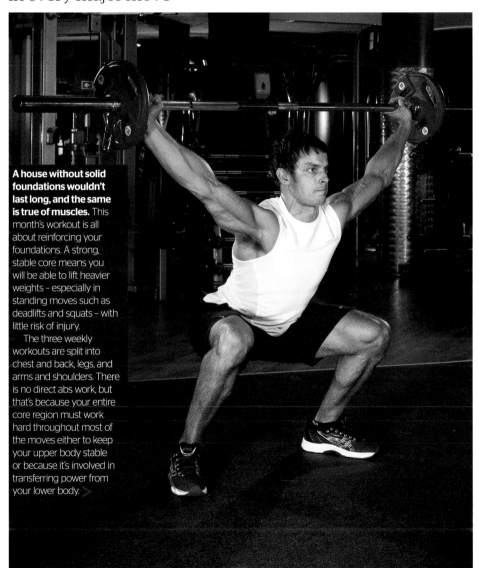

How you do it

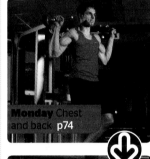
Monday Chest and back **p74**

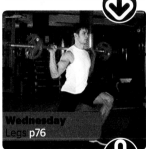
Wednesday Legs **p76**

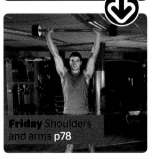
Friday Shoulders and arms **p78**

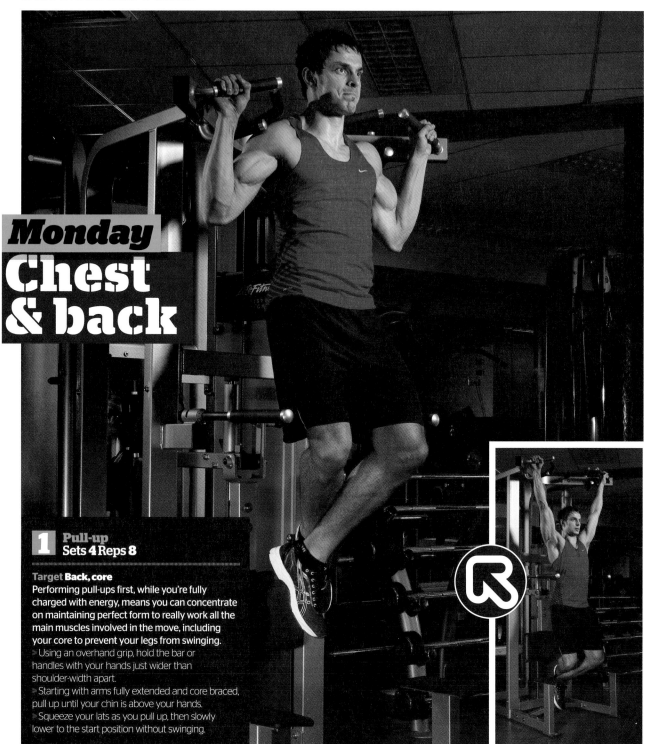

Monday
Chest & back

1 Pull-up
Sets 4 Reps 8

Target Back, core

Performing pull-ups first, while you're fully charged with energy, means you can concentrate on maintaining perfect form to really work all the main muscles involved in the move, including your core to prevent your legs from swinging.

▸ Using an overhand grip, hold the bar or handles with your hands just wider than shoulder-width apart.

▸ Starting with arms fully extended and core braced, pull up until your chin is above your hands.

▸ Squeeze your lats as you pull up, then slowly lower to the start position without swinging.

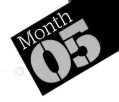

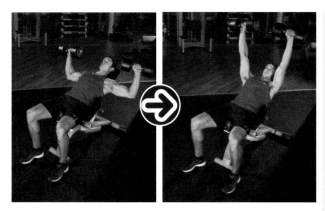

2 | Incline dumb-bell bench press
Sets 3 Reps 12

Target Chest, shoulders, triceps
This involves the shoulders more than the classic bench press does, while using dumb-bells means you do not rely on your dominant side.
> Lie on a bench with a 45° incline.
> Hold a dumb-bell in each hand at shoulder height.
> Push the weights up. Pause briefly before your arms lock out.
> Slowly lower back to the start.

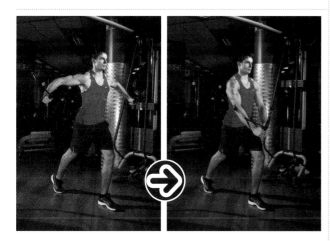

4 | Cable crossover
Sets 3 Reps 12

Target Chest
Using the cable makes your chest work hard throughout.
> Hold a D-handle cable attachment in each hand with your arms wide but elbows slightly bent.
> Stand with core braced and a natural arch in your back with your feet in a split stance.
> Bring the handles down in front of you so they cross near your navel. Squeeze your pecs for a second, then slowly return to the start.

3 | Barbell upright row
Sets 4 Reps 8

Target Back, shoulders
This move blitzes the deltoids and lats while bringing your traps into play. Using the barbell allows you to go heavy while working your core to stabilise your torso.
> Hold the bar at thigh height with an overhand grip and your hands slightly narrower than shoulder-width apart.
> With shoulders back and a natural arch in your back, shrug and pull the bar upwards, leading with your elbows until it's at shoulder height.
> Slowly return to the start.

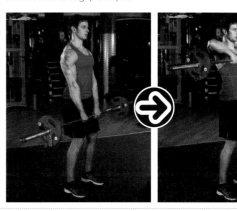

5 | Standing cable row
Sets 3 Reps 12

Target Back
This variation of the seated row keeps the emphasis on your back muscles, rather than your biceps, and engages your core throughout.
> Stand with feet shoulder-width apart holding a wide bar with an overhand grip, arms straight and leaning back until you feel resistance.
> Pull the bar towards you, leading with your elbows. Try to keep your body stationary throughout.
> Return slowly to the start.

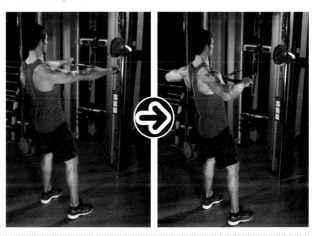

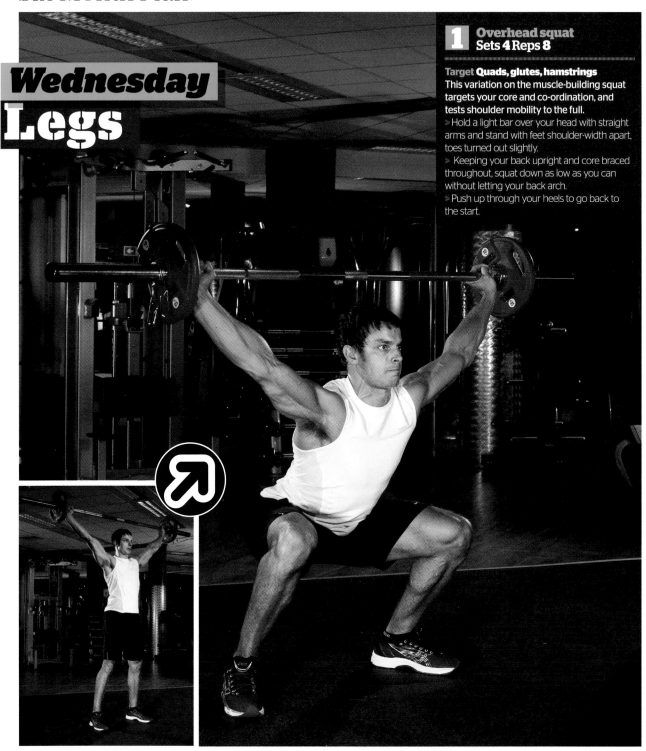

Wednesday
Legs

1 **Overhead squat**
Sets 4 Reps 8

Target Quads, glutes, hamstrings
This variation on the muscle-building squat targets your core and co-ordination, and tests shoulder mobility to the full.
› Hold a light bar over your head with straight arms and stand with feet shoulder-width apart, toes turned out slightly.
› Keeping your back upright and core braced throughout, squat down as low as you can without letting your back arch.
› Push up through your heels to go back to the start.

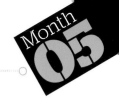

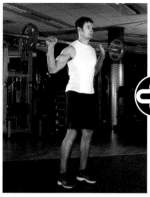

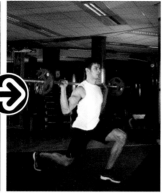

2 Lunge
Sets 3 Reps 12 each side

Target Quads, hamstrings
The lunge requires a solid core and good balance. It isolates each leg to build equal strength on both sides.
> Rest the bar across the back of your shoulders, not on your neck. Keep a natural arch in your back and core braced throughout.
> Take a big stride forward, lowering your back knee until it almost touches the floor and keeping your front knee above your front foot.
> Push off your front foot to return to the start. Swap legs.

3 One-leg Romanian deadlift
Sets 3 Reps 8 each side

Target Hamstrings
This deadlift variation works each leg hard to build strength, stability and balance. Keep good form to protect your back.
> Hold the bar with an overhand grip and each hand just outside your hips. Keep a natural arch in your back and your head up throughout.
> Standing on one leg, slowly lean forward from the hips, not the waist, and allow the bar to travel down your standing shin until you feel a good stretch in your hamstring.
> Return to the start position.

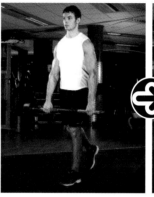

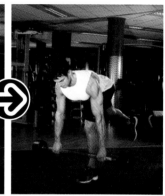

5 45° leg press
Sets 3 Reps 12

Target Quads, glutes, hamstrings
An ideal finisher – go heavy to wear out your leg muscles.
> With your back supported in the seat, place your feet on the platform.
> Engage your core, push the platform away and release the dock lever.
> Slowly lower the weight again by bending your knees.

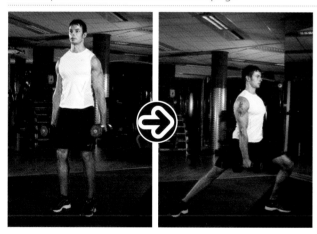

4 Transverse lunge
Sets 3 Reps 12

Target Adductors, core
This strengthens your inner thighs, which are vital in turning movements during sport.
> Stand with your feet close together, holding dumb-bells.
> Sidestep and turn your foot to 90° to the other, keeping your front knee over your foot.
> Lean on your leading leg to lower, staying upright throughout, then return to the start.

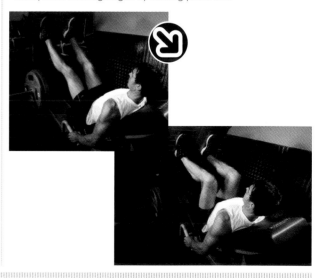

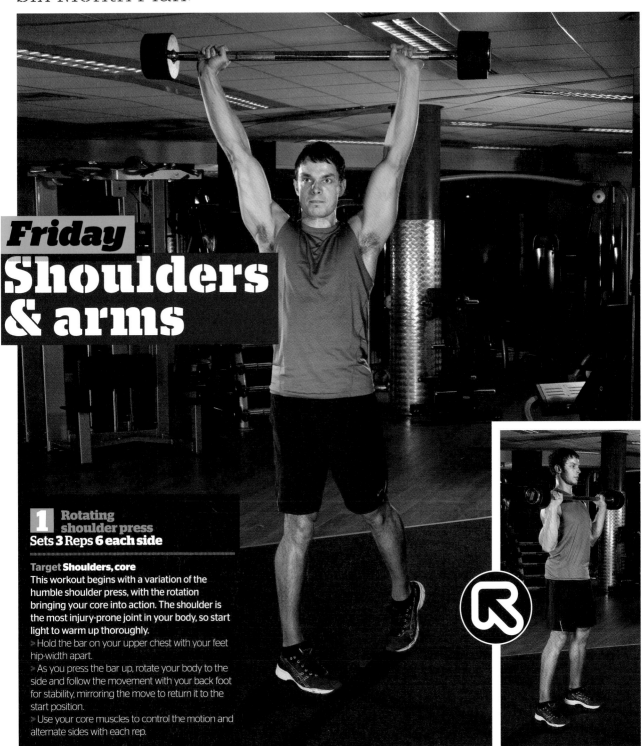

Friday
Shoulders & arms

1 Rotating shoulder press
Sets 3 Reps 6 each side

Target Shoulders, core

This workout begins with a variation of the humble shoulder press, with the rotation bringing your core into action. The shoulder is the most injury-prone joint in your body, so start light to warm up thoroughly.

> Hold the bar on your upper chest with your feet hip-width apart.

> As you press the bar up, rotate your body to the side and follow the movement with your back foot for stability, mirroring the move to return it to the start position.

> Use your core muscles to control the motion and alternate sides with each rep.

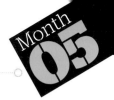

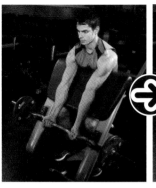
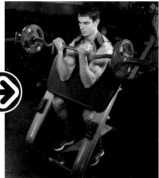

2 EZ-bar preacher curl
Sets 4 Reps 8

Target Biceps
The bench stabilises your upper arms, meaning your biceps can handle more weight so the move breaks down as many muscle fibres as possible so that they grow back stronger.

> Sit at a preacher bench and hold the bar underhand.
> Keeping your torso against the bench, curl the bar up.
> At the top, squeeze your biceps muscles, then slowly lower the bar back down.

4 Bench dip
Sets 3 Reps 12

Target Triceps
This simply blasts your arm muscles. If you find it too easy, you can rest a weight plate on your lap for faster gains.

> Sit across two parallel benches slightly less than a leg's length apart.
> Using your arms to support you, lower your body until your arms make a right angle.
> Push back up to return to the start.

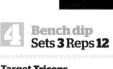

3 Alternating wide shoulder press
Sets 3 Reps 10 each side

Target Shoulders
This exercise hits your deltoid muscles from a different angle to work more muscle fibres. Like most of the other exercises here, it also involves the core for added stability.

> Stand with feet hip-width apart and hold a light dumb-bell in each hand by your shoulders.
> Keeping your core braced and without swinging your arms, raise one weight out to the side until your arms is straight and at a 45° angle to the body. Keep the other arm still throughout.
> Slowly return to the start, alternating arms with each rep.

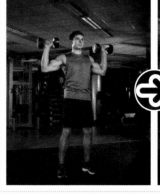
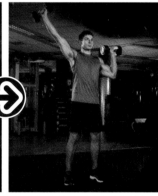

5 Diagonal cable raise Sets 3
Sets 2 Reps 10 each side

Target Shoulders
This move fatigues your delts and also works the stabilising muscles.
> Attach a stirrup handle to the low pulley of a cable station. Stand side-on to it, holding the handle so your arm goes across your body.
> With core engaged and legs straight, pull the cable up and across your body until your hand is above your head. Slowly return to the start.

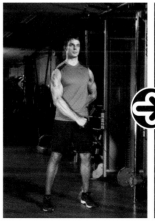
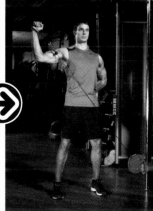

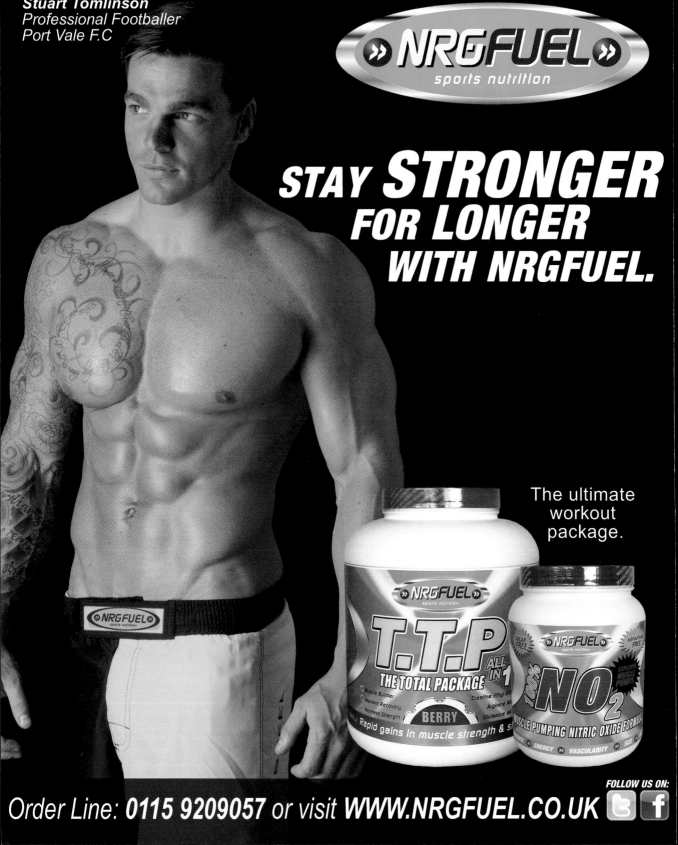

Month
06

Aim for the top

Hit your upper body this month and reveal your six-pack

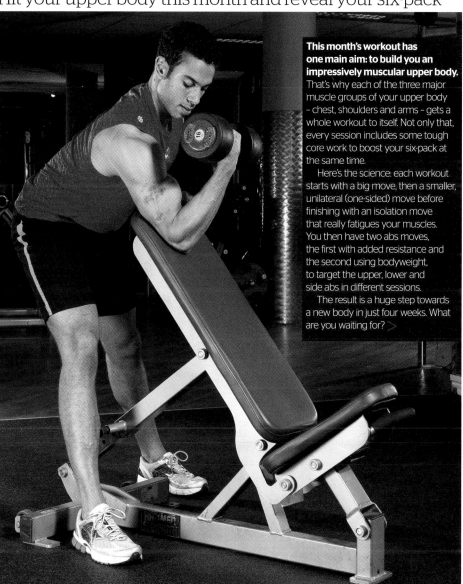

This month's workout has one main aim: to build you an impressively muscular upper body. That's why each of the three major muscle groups of your upper body – chest, shoulders and arms – gets a whole workout to itself. Not only that, every session includes some tough core work to boost your six-pack at the same time.

Here's the science: each workout starts with a big move, then a smaller, unilateral (one-sided) move before finishing with an isolation move that really fatigues your muscles. You then have two abs moves, the first with added resistance and the second using bodyweight, to target the upper, lower and side abs in different sessions.

The result is a huge step towards a new body in just four weeks. What are you waiting for? ▶

How to do it

 Timing Workouts should take about 30 minutes, including the warm-up.

 Warm-up Spend five minutes doing bodyweight moves such as press-ups, squats and lunges.

 Weight Choose a weight that allows you to complete all your reps but no more.

 Tempo Take one second to lift the weight, pause, then take three seconds to lower.

 Rest Rest for 30-45 seconds between sets and for one minute between exercises.

How you do it

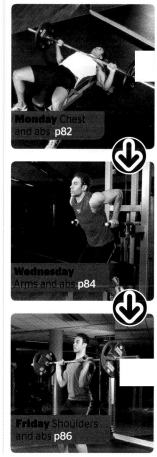

Monday Chest and abs **p82**

Wednesday Arms and abs **p84**

Friday Shoulders and abs **p86**

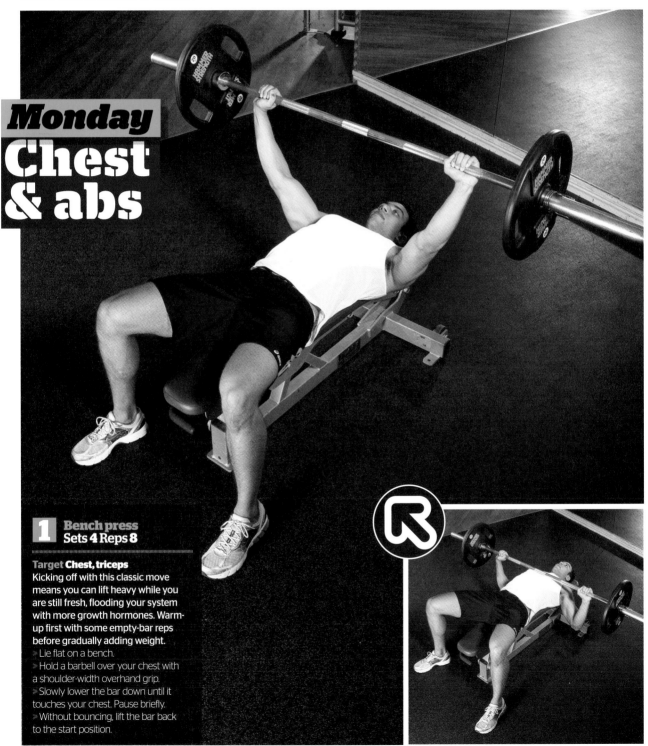

Monday
Chest & abs

1 Bench press
Sets 4 Reps 8

Target Chest, triceps
Kicking off with this classic move means you can lift heavy while you are still fresh, flooding your system with more growth hormones. Warm-up first with some empty-bar reps before gradually adding weight.
> Lie flat on a bench.
> Hold a barbell over your chest with a shoulder-width overhand grip.
> Slowly lower the bar down until it touches your chest. Pause briefly.
> Without bouncing, lift the bar back to the start position.

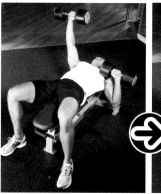
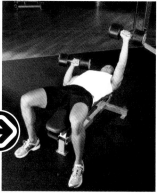

2 Alternating dumb-bell bench press
Sets 3 Reps 8 each side

Target Chest, triceps
With the target muscles now firing, you hit them hard again with this single-arm move. Using one arm at a time allows you to correct any muscular imbalances and makes your core work harder for longer.
> Lie flat on a bench with a dumb-bell in each hand just by your shoulders.
> Press one weight up until your arm is almost fully extended.
> Slowly lower it back down, then press up with the other arm.

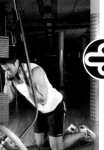
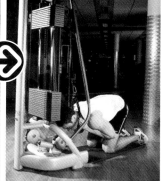

4 Kneeling cable crunch
Sets 3 Reps 15

Target Upper abs
Working your abs with additional resistance, such as that on the cable stack, is a surefire way of forcing them into growing bigger and stronger.
> With the double-rope attachment secured to the top of the cable machine, kneel down facing the weight stack.

> Hold a rope in each hand on either side of your head.
> Slowly crunch your torso forward and down towards the floor.
> Once your back is parallel to the floor, pause briefly, then return slowly to the top.

3 Gym ball dumb-bell flye
Sets 4 Reps 6-8

Target Chest
To really fatigue the chest muscles, perform this isolation move. Since your muscles will be tired, start with light dumb-bells – you can always go heavier if the first set is too easy.
> Lie with your back on a gym ball, holding a dumb-bell in each hand

directly above your chest.
> Keeping your core braced and a slight bend in your elbows, slowly lower your hands down and out to the side until you feel a stretch across your chest. Pause briefly, then return to the top.

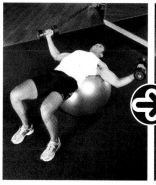
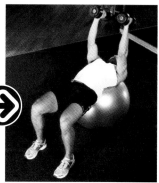

5 Gym ball crunch
Sets 3 Reps To failure

Target Upper abs
Almost done. All that's left is to finish off your abs with this twist on the classic crunch. Using a gym ball provides a greater range of motion for your abs to work through, resulting in more gains.

> Lie with your back over a gym ball.
> With your fingers at your temples, crunch up.
> Pause briefly at the top of the move then slowly lower back to the start. Pause there, then repeat.

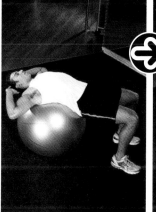
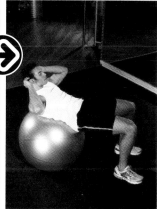

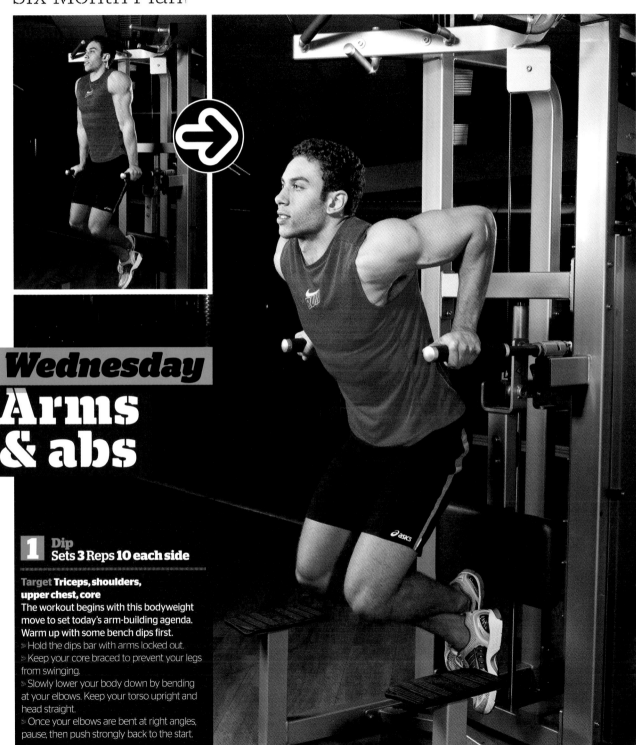

Wednesday

Arms & abs

1 Dip
Sets 3 Reps 10 each side

Target Triceps, shoulders, upper chest, core

The workout begins with this bodyweight move to set today's arm-building agenda. Warm up with some bench dips first.

▷ Hold the dips bar with arms locked out.

▷ Keep your core braced to prevent your legs from swinging.

▷ Slowly lower your body down by bending at your elbows. Keep your torso upright and head straight.

▷ Once your elbows are bent at right angles, pause, then push strongly back to the start.

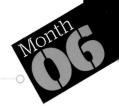

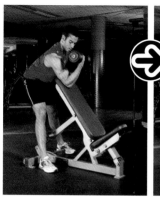
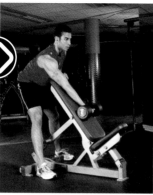

2 One-arm preacher curl
Sets 3 Reps 10 each side

Target Biceps
Next up are the biceps. Working one arm at a time over a bench allows you to go heavy while not allowing you to use momentum. Your biceps have no option but to do all the work.
> Stand behind a bench set at about 60°.

> Hold a dumb-bell in one hand fully extended down the front of the bench.
> Keeping your upper arm flush against the bench, slowly curl the weight up.
> Once at the top, squeeze your biceps, then slowly lower the weight back down.

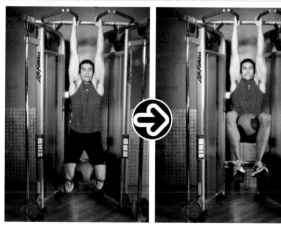

4 Hanging medicine ball knee raise
Sets 3 Reps 8

Target Lower abs
Knee raises are great for hitting the lower abs. Additional weight from a medicine ball makes them far harder for greater results.
> Hang from a pull-up bar with a medicine ball held securely

between your knees.
> Keeping your upper body stable, slowly draw your knees up towards your chest.
> Pause for a second, then slowly return your legs to the start position.

3 Seated one-arm overhead triceps extension
Sets 3 Reps 10 each side

Target Triceps, core
It's time to return to your triceps, which make up the largest part of your upper arm musculature. Isolating them damages the muscle fibres, which will then grow back bigger.
> Sit on a bench holding a dumb-bell in one hand directly above your head.
> Lower the weight behind your head by bending at the elbow.
> Pause briefly, then straighten your arm to return the weight back to the top.

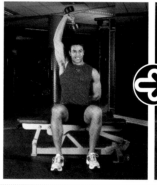
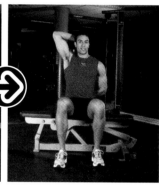

5 Bench V-sit
Sets 3 Reps To failure

Target Chest
Because it's the last move of this workout and one with minimum risk, perform this lower-abs move to failure on each set to really blitz your muscles for maximum reward.
> Sit on a bench and lean back with your feet off the floor. Grip the side of

the bench with your hands for support.
> Slowly draw your knees into your chest, pause briefly, then return them out in front of you.
> Keep your feet off the floor throughout the set to work your lower abs more thoroughly.

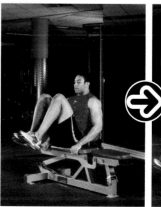
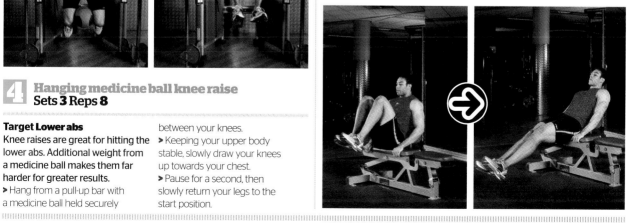

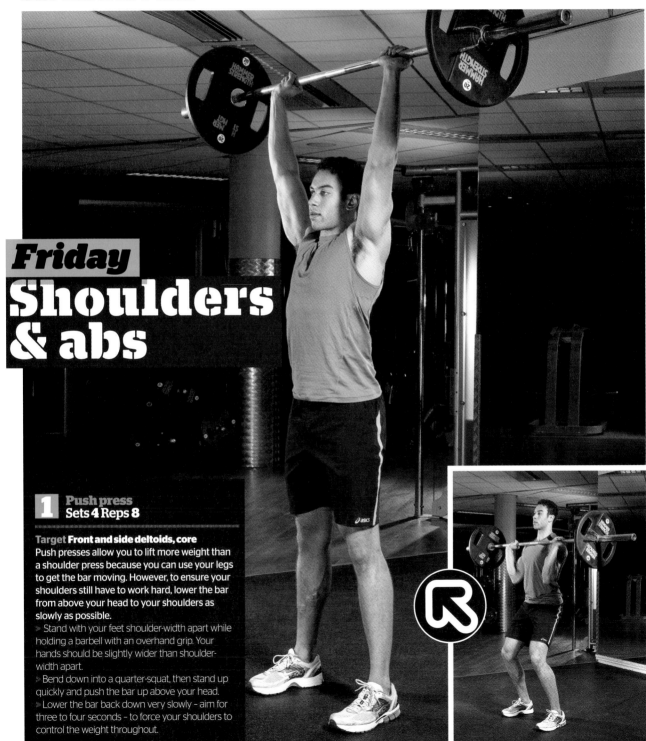

Friday
Shoulders & abs

1 Push press
Sets 4 Reps 8

Target Front and side deltoids, core

Push presses allow you to lift more weight than a shoulder press because you can use your legs to get the bar moving. However, to ensure your shoulders still have to work hard, lower the bar from above your head to your shoulders as slowly as possible.

> Stand with your feet shoulder-width apart while holding a barbell with an overhand grip. Your hands should be slightly wider than shoulder-width apart.

> Bend down into a quarter-squat, then stand up quickly and push the bar up above your head.

> Lower the bar back down very slowly – aim for three to four seconds – to force your shoulders to control the weight throughout.

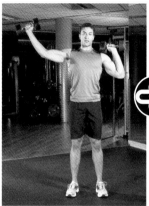 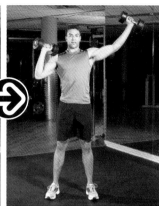

2 Dumb-bell alternating wide shoulder press
Sets 3 Reps 8 each side

Target Front and side deltoids
A slight twist turns the humble shoulder press into this tough move that will build wide shoulders.

> Stand with feet hip-width apart with a dumb-bell held in each hand at shoulder height.
> One hand at a time, press the dumb-bell up and out at 45°.
> Slowly return to the start and repeat with the other arm.

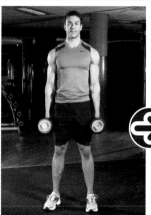 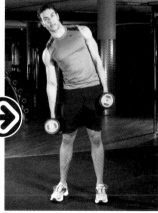

4 Dumb-bell side bend
Sets 3 Reps 12 each side

Target Obliques
This move works the hard-to-target side abs, also known as the obliques. Again, the small range of motion allows you to go for heavy dumb-bells.

> Stand with feet hip-width apart, holding a dumb-bell in each hand.
> Slowly bend from the hips to one side as far as is comfortable, then return to the upright position.
> Repeat on the other side.

3 Shrug
Sets 4 Reps 12

Target Traps
Shrugs are great for building big traps. This move has a small range of motion so you can go heavy.

> Stand with feet hip-width apart with a heavy dumb-bell in each hand.
> Keep your core braced, a natural arch in your back and slightly retract your shoulder blades.
> Shrug your shoulders up to almost ear-height. Pause at this top position and squeeze your traps for a second.
> Lower back to the start.

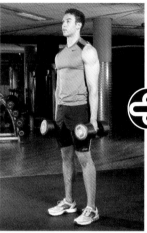 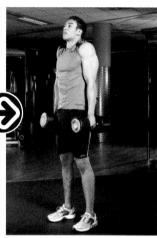

5 Gym ball oblique crunch
Sets 3 Reps 12 each side

Target Triceps
Finish off the session by again hitting the obliques.

> Lie with one side on a gym ball. Place your fingers by your temples.
> Crunch up by contracting your abs.
> Pause briefly at the top, then slowly return to the start.

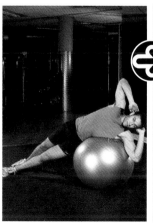 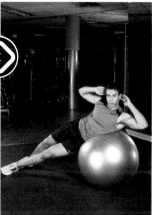

10 six-pack foods

You might have the world's most well-sculpted abs, but unless you burn off the fat that covers them you won't be displaying a six-pack. These foods should help

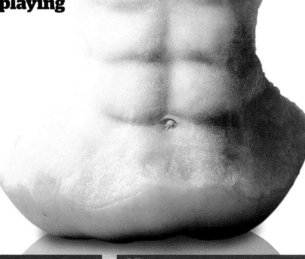

1 Apples

You'll get at least 5g of fibre from one large apple, which helps you feel full. US research discovered that people who ate a large apple 15 minutes before lunch took in 190 fewer calories during lunch than those who didn't snack beforehand. This is because apples are nearly 85 per cent water and require lots of chewing, which can make you feel like you are eating more than you are.

➤ **1 apple** Calories **47** Carbs **11.8g** Protein **0.4g** Fat **0.1g**

For a healthy dessert chop and bake in the oven with cinnamon

2 Cottage cheese

This protein-rich food is brimming with casein, a protein that is digested slowly and provides the body with long-lasting energy. Research from the Netherlands also found that people with a diet high in casein increased their metabolism, their satiety levels and their body's use of fat.

➤ **150g** Calories **128** Carbs **5.1g** Protein **21.5g** Fat **2.3g**

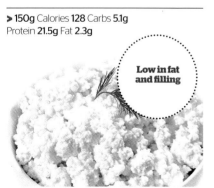

Low in fat and filling

3 Asparagus

This nutrient powerhouse contains chromium to control blood sugar levels and banish cravings. It also has vitamins K and C, which boost calcium absorption and metabolism. It may also reduce excess oestrogen in the body, which in turn helps the body's ability to use fat stores for energy.

➤ **4 spears** Calories **13** Carbs **2g** Protein **1g** Fat **0g**

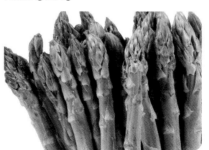

4 Beans

Every schoolboy knows beans are good for your heart. And they're good for your abs: rich in fibre, potassium (to balance blood sugar), protein and testosterone-boosting zinc. A US survey found that people who ate beans were 23 per cent less likely to have large waists than those who didn't.

➤ **1 heaped tbsp** Calories **91** Carbs **13.9g** Protein **6.4g** Fat **1.5g**

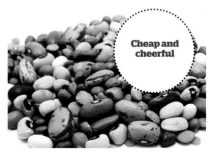

Cheap and cheerful

5 Grapefruit

The grapefruit diet was just a fad like any other – but there are definite advantages to eating the fruit. In a study, people who ate half a grapefruit with each meal lost an average of 1.6kg in three months. This is because grapefruits lower your post-meal levels of insulin, the hormone that regulates blood sugar and fat metabolism.

➤ Half a grapefruit Calories 41
Carbs 10.3g Protein 0.8g Fat 0.1g

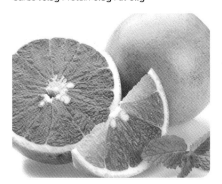

6 Olive oil

You may think you should avoid oils when you're trying to lose fat, but the oleic acid in olive oil can give you a helping hand. According to an American study in the journal Cell Metabolism, it can squash appetite because it's converted into a compound called oleoylethanololamide (OEA) that indirectly triggers hunger-curbing signals to your brain.

➤ 1tsp Calories 40 Carbs 0g
Protein 0g Fat 4.5g

Spritz olive oil instead of drizzling when cooking

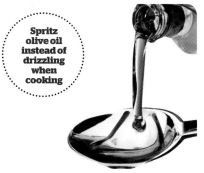

7 Potato

The low-carb craze led people to think you couldn't eat potatoes and lose weight, but they contain starch, which resists digestion and keeps you fuller for longer. Danish studies have also found that starch can improve blood-sugar control, which helps the body burn fat. Eat them chilled to get nearly double the starch from each one.

➤ 110g Calories 75 Carbs 17.1g
Protein 1.7g Fat 0.3g

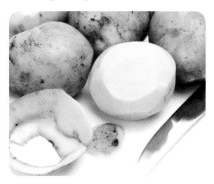

8 Rocket

Rocket is ideal fat loss food – low in calories, high in fibre and rich in calcium, an essential mineral for muscle contraction. It also contains glucosinolates, nutrients that eliminate harmful toxins in the body. And since it's in the mustard family rather than a type of lettuce, rocket has a strong, peppery flavour that means your salads won't be bland.

➤ 50g Calories 10 Carbs 1.1g
Protein 0.7g Fat 0.3g

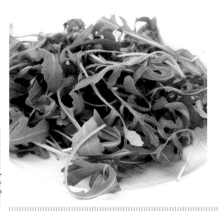

9 Almonds

Nuts are high in fat but aren't fattening. Instead, research shows the composition of their cell walls may help reduce the absorption of all their fat, so they provide fewer calories than would be expected. They are also a good source of magnesium, which helps produce energy, maintain muscle tissue and regulate blood sugar levels.

➤ 24 almonds Calories 163 Carbs 6.1g Protein 6g
Fat 14g

Long lasting: buy in bulk

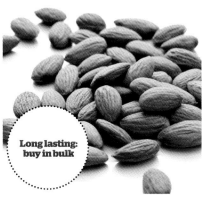

10 Iced coffee

Studies have shown caffeine to reduce appetite and increase metabolism. It blocks the production in the brain of a chemical called adenosine, which makes you feel fatigued and susceptible to pain, so you can work out harder for longer. Make your own iced coffee by brewing up, allowing it to cool then blending with ice cubes and a splash of milk.

➤ 1 glass Calories 35 Carbs 4g
Protein 2g Fat 1g

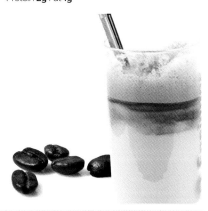

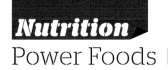

Nutrition

Power Foods

Eat to build muscle

Get the energy you need for serious weight training with these ideal meals

Breakfast

Porridge and berries Mix 50g oats with milk. Boil for five minutes and stir frequently. Serve with blueberries, chopped almonds and 1tsp honey

> Oats are full of slow-digesting carbs that will give you enough energy to get you through the day.
> The vitamin C in the blueberries can help lower cortisol, a hormone associated with muscle breakdown.
> Honey is an instant energy booster, which can also help lower blood sugar levels as well as reducing muscle and joint inflammation.
> Almonds will keep your levels of good fats high. They also have anti-inflammatory properties, to keep your joints supple and healthy.

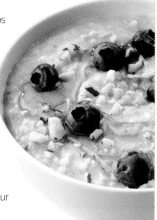

Morning snack

Toast and shake 50g cheddar cheese toasted on 2 slices of wholemeal bread and a protein shake made with 200ml semi-skimmed milk

> While low in fat, the cheese is high in protein and calcium.
> Milk contains protein, calcium and the amino acid leucine, which together build muscle and promote fat-burning.
> The whey in the protein shake is rich in the proteins your body uses to make testosterone, the muscle-building hormone.

WHEN YOU WAKE... your muscles are primed to take in large amounts of calories (especially carbs) without inducing high levels of fat storage. Breakfast will also boost your metabolism, helping you burn fat for the rest of the day.

Lunch

Sandwich and soup
Turkey, spinach and avocado wholemeal baguette and 1 can of tomato soup

> Spinach will strengthen your bones thanks to its vitamin K content, which helps the body process calcium. It is also packed with iron, an essential mineral that controls the release of energy.
> Avocado is full of essential fats, which the body needs to absorb fat-soluble vitamins and store glucose as muscle glycogen.
> The wholemeal bread is full of slow-releasing carbs, which you need to fuel your muscles with glycogen.
> Soup is virtually fat-free yet full of antioxidants, which may help to reduce muscle soreness and ward off age-related diseases.

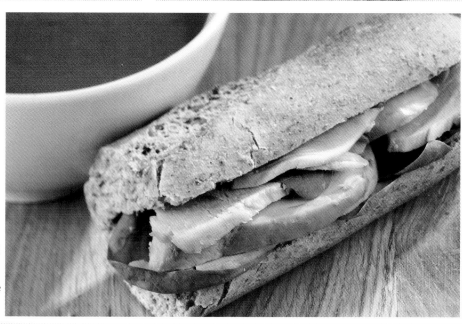

Pre-workout snack

Crunchy biscuits Peanut butter on 2 oatcakes and cinnamon herbal supplement

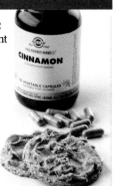

> Peanut butter is a great source of slow-release energy that will drip-feed your muscles as you work out.
> The fibre in the oatcakes will fill you up so you don't feel peckish mid-workout.
> Cinnamon can help regulate blood sugar levels, which will keep your energy up throughout the day and get rid of post-training sugar cravings. See solgar-vitamins.co.uk.

Post-workout snack

Muesli, berries and yoghurt with a creatine shake Blend 75g natural yoghurt with 25g muesli, 60g strawberries and 20g hazelnuts. 10g creatine powder with 400ml water

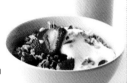

> Yoghurt contains protein, calcium and vitamin B12.
> Your body uses the vitamin C from the strawberries to aid muscle recovery.
> To avoid energy slumps, eat carbs after exercise. The oats and grains in muesli will replace muscle glycogen.
> Creatine helps reduce protein breakdown following exercise and can aid recovery.

Dinner

Grilled tuna steak with baked sweet potato
With a side salad with a squeeze of lemon juice

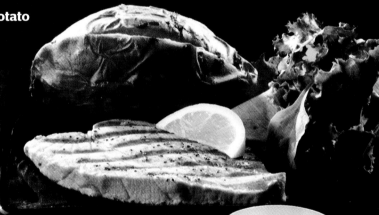

> One sweet potato has about 10 per cent of your daily recommended allowance of potassium, a mineral your body needs for normal muscle function.
> Tuna is rich in coenzyme Q10, which gives you energy, vitamin A and zinc for testosterone, and protein to rebuild muscle and torn fibres.
> Squeezing lemon juice over your greens will enhance iron absorption, while a selection of lettuce leaves will supply you with phytonutrients – plant-derived nutrients that will keep you fighting fit.

Pre-bed snack

Peanut butter and banana smoothie
Blend 1tbsp peanut butter, 150-200ml semi-skimmed milk, ½ a banana, 1tbsp sesame seeds and 1tsp linseeds

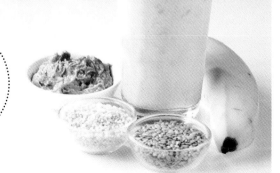

> The high protein content of peanut butter will feed your muscles and make you feel full, so you won't wake up with an attack of midnight munchies.
> Bananas have a high magnesium content to help relax and repair your muscles.
> Calcium-rich milk helps the brain use the sleep-inducing amino acid tryptophan and produce melatonin, which regulates your sleep cycle.
> Linseeds are packed with omega 3 fatty acids and fibre, which helps detoxify your gut while you sleep.

YOUR MUSCLES NEED nutrients to regenerate while you sleep, so eat an hour before bed if you're trying to bulk up.

TOTALS > 2,909 calories > 270g carbs > 189g protein > 92g fat

Protein sweets

You don't have to always take your muscle-gain powder in the form of a shake. These sweet snacks will give your protein a tasty twist

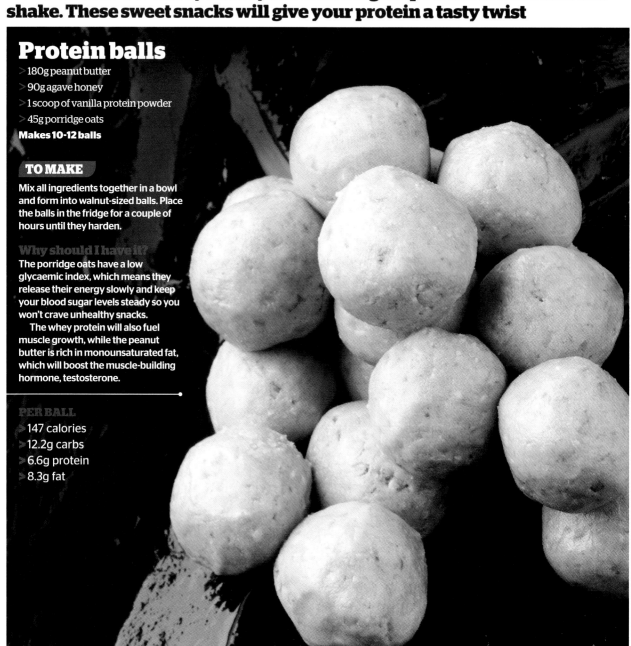

Protein balls

> 180g peanut butter
> 90g agave honey
> 1 scoop of vanilla protein powder
> 45g porridge oats

Makes 10-12 balls

TO MAKE

Mix all ingredients together in a bowl and form into walnut-sized balls. Place the balls in the fridge for a couple of hours until they harden.

Why should I have it?

The porridge oats have a low glycaemic index, which means they release their energy slowly and keep your blood sugar levels steady so you won't crave unhealthy snacks.

The whey protein will also fuel muscle growth, while the peanut butter is rich in monounsaturated fat, which will boost the muscle-building hormone, testosterone.

PER BALL

> 147 calories
> 12.2g carbs
> 6.6g protein
> 8.3g fat

Apricot and almond bar

- 3 large oranges with pips removed
- 170g almond butter
- 350g dried apricots, chopped
- 225g porridge oats
- 1 scoop of vanilla protein powder
- 125g wholemeal self-raising flour
- 25g mixed seeds
- ½tsp bicarbonate of soda
- 1tsp ground cinnamon

Makes 16 bars

TO MAKE

Preheat the oven to 190˚C (Gas Mark 5). Measure 225g of the dried apricots and purée them with the oranges and almond butter in a blender to form a thick paste.

Place the oats, flour, seeds, protein powder, soda and cinnamon in a large bowl. Stir in the rest of the apricots and then combine with the purée.

Press the mixture into a greased shallow rectangular tin and smooth the top with the back of a spoon. Bake in the oven for 20-25 minutes until golden brown. Leave to cool for ten minutes, then cut into small bars and store in an airtight container in the fridge.

Why should I have it?

The nut butter and seeds are full of muscle-building protein, while the oats provide the B vitamins needed for efficient energy release. Cinnamon contains anti-inflammatory compounds that soothe stiff muscles, while bicarbonate of soda can reduce lactic acid production in muscles, meaning you can train for longer.

PER BAR > 202 calories > 25.1g carbs > 7.8g protein > 8.4g fat

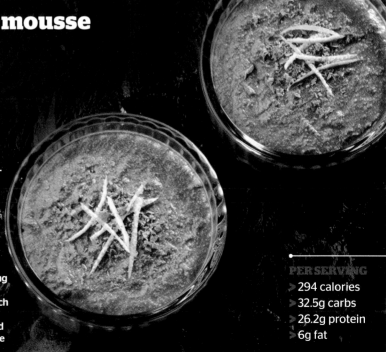

Chocolate & orange mousse

- 175g plain chocolate (75 per cent cocoa solids)
- 350g silken tofu
- 1 scoop of chocolate protein powder
- Juice and zest of 2 oranges
- Grated orange zest and chocolate, to serve

Serves 4

TO MAKE

Melt the chocolate in a bowl over a pan of simmering water, stirring occasionally. Allow to cool slightly. Place the tofu, protein powder and orange zest and juice in a food processor or blender and blend until smooth and creamy.

Spoon into four individual dishes and chill in the fridge until set. Decorate with a little orange zest and grated chocolate.

Why should I have it?

Known for their muscle-healing vitamin C content, oranges are also packed with photochemical and flavonoids that protect muscles from oxidative damage caused by exercise. Tofu also contains muscle-building protein and calcium, as well as isoflavones, which can block the female hormone oestrogen and make testosterone more prevalent.

PER SERVING
- 294 calories
- 32.5g carbs
- 26.2g protein
- 6g fat

Mammoth appetite

Eat like a caveman to add power to your workouts and prevent weight gain

For thousands of years, humans had no refined sugars or processed foods. So although such modern grub may be tasty and convenient, your body hasn't evolved to deal with it very well – and it usually encourages fat storage. This meal plan, created by nutritionist Christine Bailey (advancenutrition.co.uk) and based on the Paleo Diet for Athletes, replaces processed sugary foods and carbs with fresh fruit, nuts, seeds and animal proteins – the staple Stone Age foods. It has plenty of healthy unsaturated fats and branched-chain amino acids, which as well as aiding fat loss will help muscle development and anabolic function.

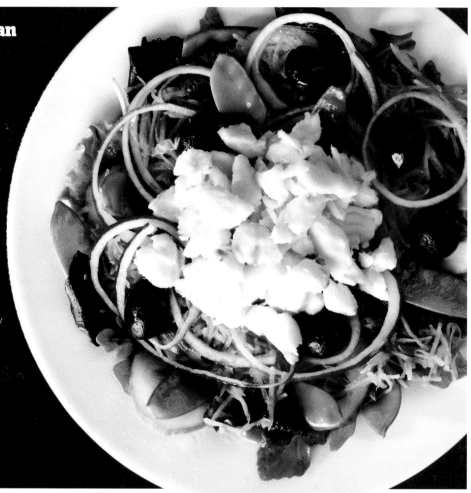

Lemon crab salad

To make
Mix 1 bag of mixed salad leaves, ½ a sliced red onion, a handful of black olives, some cucumber slices, sugar snap peas and 1 grated carrot. Top with a 125g can of white crab meat and dress with lemon juice and olive oil.

Red onion
contains fat-melting vitamin C and chromium, a mineral that helps insulin response, stopping sugar cravings.

Carrots
are high in the soluble fibre calcium pectate. This fills you up and binds with acids in the body to reduce cholesterol levels.

Crab meat
is low in fat and calories but rich in omega 3 fatty acids, which can reduce hunger pangs and help muscle growth.

Olives
have omega 3 fatty acids that trigger hunger-curbing signals in your brain. They are also rich in vitamins A, C and E.

Photography foodanddrinkphotos.com

42 prehistoric meals that will keep the flab at bay

Monday	Tuesday	Wednesday	Thursday	Friday	Saturday	Sunday
Breakfast 1 grapefruit. 2-egg omelette with ½ an avocado, spinach and 2 chopped tomatoes.	**Breakfast** 150g sautéed prawns with 6 sliced mushrooms and ½ chopped red pepper. 150g fresh pineapple slices.	**Breakfast** Bowl of blueberries and raspberries. 2 poached eggs with asparagus and 4 grilled mushrooms.	**Breakfast** Slices of melon with cashew nuts. 3 slices of lean roast beef with 2 baked tomatoes.	**Breakfast** Bowl of cherries. 2 scrambled eggs with 5 asparagus spears.	**Breakfast** Bowl of blueberries and raspberries. 1 cold salmon fillet with pan-fried tomatoes and mushrooms.	**Breakfast** 100g cooked prawns with green beans. 1 chopped apple and 2tbsp seeds.
Snack 1 banana.	**Snack** Smoked salmon slices. Carrot and celery sticks.	**Snack** Handful of seeds. 1 apple.	**Snack** 1 apple. Handful of raisins and almonds.	**Snack** 2 slices of ham, sliced cucumber and celery.	**Snack** 4 oatcakes with ham.	**Snack** 2 slices of ham and 2 tomatoes.
Lunch 150g grilled cod fillet with lemon juice and freshly ground black pepper. Green salad with lemon juice and 1tsp olive oil, 50g sugar snap peas, cucumber slices, ½ a red pepper and 2tbsp black olives. Bowl of blueberries and melon.	**Lunch** Chicken and avocado salad. 1 apple. 30g almonds.	**Lunch** ½ a carton of Covent Garden Tomato & Basil soup. Cold venison steak served with a bag of mixed salad leaves, ½ red pepper, 2tbsp black olives, sliced cucumber, celery and 1 tomato. Slices of melon.	**Lunch** 300ml Covent Garden Scotch Broth soup. Grilled pork fillet with spinach salad (handful of baby spinach leaves, mixed lettuce leaves, ½ red onion, ½ red pepper, chopped fresh cucumber slices, celery). 1 satsuma.	**Lunch** Leftover squash and turkey casserole. Large mixed salad.	**Lunch** Grilled turkey breast with 1 baked sweet potato, salad leaves, cucumber, sugar snap peas, ½ a red pepper, 2tbsp black olives and ½ a red onion. Slices of fresh pineapple.	**Lunch** Lemon crab salad (see recipe). Slices of melon.
Snack 3 cold lean beef slices. Carrot sticks.	**Snack** 1 hard-boiled egg. 2 oatcakes.	**Snack** 2 slices of ham. Carrot sticks.	**Snack** 1 hard-boiled egg. Carrot sticks.	**Snack** Handful of raisins and almonds. 1 pear.	**Snack** 100g cooked prawns. Celery and carrot sticks.	**Snack** 2 oatcakes. Smoked salmon slices.
Dinner Ginger baked turkey. 100g fresh raspberries with 2tbsp flaked almonds.	**Dinner** 300ml Covent Garden Scotch Broth soup. Pan-fried venison with cherry sauce.	**Dinner** Chicken cashew nut stir-fry. Sliced fresh pineapple.	**Dinner** Baked butternut squash and turkey casserole.	**Dinner** 300ml Covent Garden Tomato & Basil soup. Baked salmon fillet with lemon juice (cook an extra salmon fillet for Sat) served with 60g steamed carrots, 60g sugar snap peas, 60g green beans and 1 baked sweet potato.	**Dinner** Frittata made with 2 eggs, 3 new potatoes, spinach leaves and 1 red pepper. Steamed broccoli and carrots and salad.	**Dinner** Pork stir fry. 1 satsuma.
Snack 30g macadamia nuts. Handful of raisins.	**Snack** 2 satsumas.	**Snack** 1 banana. Handful of macadamia nuts.	**Snack** 2 oatcakes. Smoked salmon slices.	**Snack** 1 banana. Handful of cashew nuts.	**Snack** 1 banana. Handful of macadamia nuts.	**Snack** 2 oatcakes. Handful of almonds and raisins
Daily total 1,840 calories, 163g carbs, 130g protein, 79g fat	**Daily total** 1,713 calories, 147g carbs, 156g protein, 60g fat	**Daily total** 1,956 calories, 179g carbs, 130g protein, 87g fat	**Daily total** 1,841 calories, 201g carbs, 138g protein, 60g fat	**Daily total** 1,816 calories, 185g carbs, 120g protein, 71g fat	**Daily total** 1,827 calories, 172g carbs, 133g protein, 72g fat	**Daily total** 1,746 calories, 159g carbs, 140g protein, 66g fat

Be a sports superstar

Train like an athlete with workouts from the world's top sportsmen

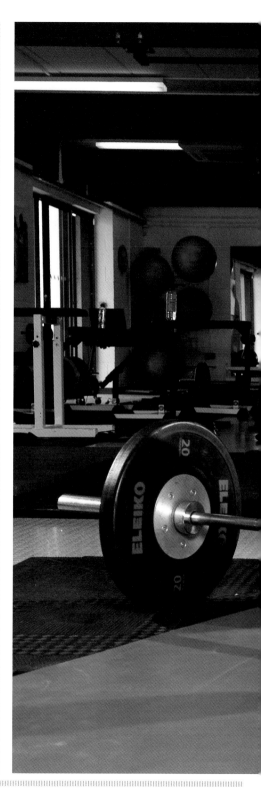

World-class sportsmen make what they do look easy. The reason they're able to make what they do look so effortless is because they spend so much time training. We've showcased sportsmen across a range of disciplines from triathlon to climbing but they all have one thing in common. The moves they do make them masters of their own bodies. All the drills in this section will help improve your co-ordination, balance and agility.

The rowing drills from Olympic gold medal winner Andrew Hodge focus on big powerful moves that build real strngth. Surf champ Romain Cloitre does explosive moves and balance training. Top triathlete Will Clarke's workouts will develop core strength, while leading climber Leo Houlding shows you how to increase your stength to weight ratio. Finally, freestyle snowboarder Marko Grilc focuses in mobility and flexibility. Do them all and you'll be better conditioned for any sport.

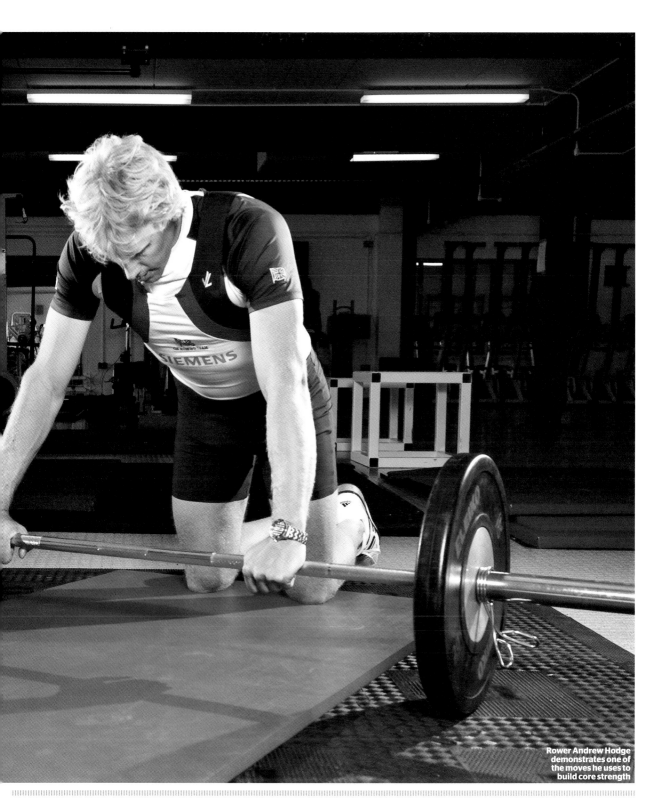

Rower Andrew Hodge demonstrates one of the moves he uses to build core strength

POWER BOAT

Find out how top British rower Andrew Hodge delivers maximum power with every stroke

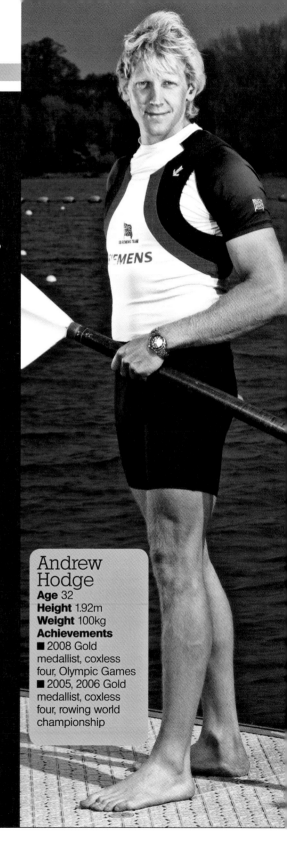

How's training going?

It's going well, thanks. Rowing's more like boxing than football and rugby. We go through long periods where we're just training, then towards competition time we go harder and start to focus more on speed work. When we're just training we'll do three sessions a day with one day off a month – it's designed to train you right on the red line.

We're also doing three or four weight sessions a week, with good steady-rate rowing on the ergo [indoor rowing machine] or on the water. It's about power and endurance, increasing both qualities.

That's a lot of training. How much do you eat?

The golden rule nutritionally is to eat enough. I think I'm at around 5,000 calories a day. Some people find it hard to keep weight on during the camps when you're training hard, but I can eat above my needs, so I try to eat healthy. You just adapt. It's about sticking to good carbs, not cheap ones, eating steadily throughout the day rather than massive meals.

Do you mainly train on the water, or on rowing machines?

Most of the time we'll try to train on the water. The ergo is good because you've got hard numbers – you can measure lactate thresholds and improve in specific areas. But you can't rely on ergo times. There are guys that aren't that great on the ergo but are great on the water, either because they've got a competition mindset or because they motivate other people really well.

How hard do you have to work on technique?

I still do technique every day. It's like a ball of putty – it's always being pushed out of shape and you want it to be perfect and round. I'm constantly addressing it, constantly trying to make it as sharp as it can be. I'll let it fall out shape in certain circumstances. Like if I've got a back niggle, I might need to let it recover by ignoring certain parts of the stroke. But then I'll need to perfect it again before an event.

You've rowed with Peter Reed since the Oxford-Cambridge boat race. How important is a good partnership?

A good understanding with your team-mate is paramount – a willingness to meet in the middle on things and discuss things openly is massively important. You need to use each other to the maximum.

> 'Technique is like a ball of putty. It's being pushed out of shape and you want it perfect and round'

Andrew Hodge

Age 32
Height 1.92m
Weight 100kg
Achievements
■ 2008 Gold medallist, coxless four, Olympic Games
■ 2005, 2006 Gold medallist, coxless four, rowing world championship

Part 1
POWER

'The key component of a good rowing stroke is delivering maximum dynamic power throughout the body,' says Hodge. 'So we'll do a lot of full-body moves that emphasise that. We also do a lot of unilateral movements. When we drive, we drive through both hips at a slightly different angle, and with the amount of strokes we do a day you can get into some real problems because of imbalances in the amount each muscle works. So it's important to balance that out in training. We'll do a lot of pushing movements for the same reason – if you work just your pulling muscles you'll end up imbalanced and injured.'

1 Split squat
Sets 3 **Reps** 5 each side

With a barbell on your back take a big step forwards, then bend your front knee until your back knee brushes the floor. Don't return to upright between reps.

Hodge says
'Don't drop your tail leg to the floor to make the move easier. You want your back in an upright, strong position.'

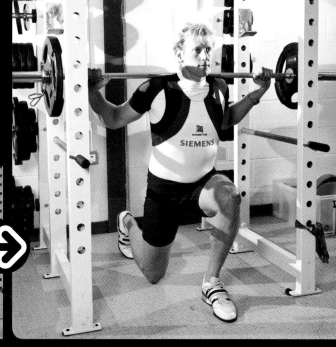

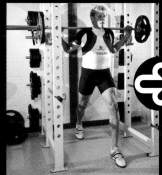

2 Power clean
Sets 5 **Reps** 3

Start with feet shoulder-width apart and grip the bar just outside your knees. Drive up and rise up on to your toes, pulling the bar upwards, then drop underneath and catch it on top of your chest. As with a rowing stroke, most of the drive should come from your legs – you shouldn't really feel this move in your arms.

Hodge says
'You want to engage your posterior chain, so stay on your heels through the drive and accelerate as you go up. As soon as your hands pass your knees, accelerate the bar up so you can drop under and catch it.'

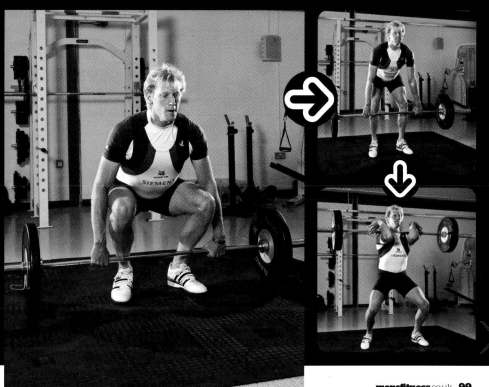

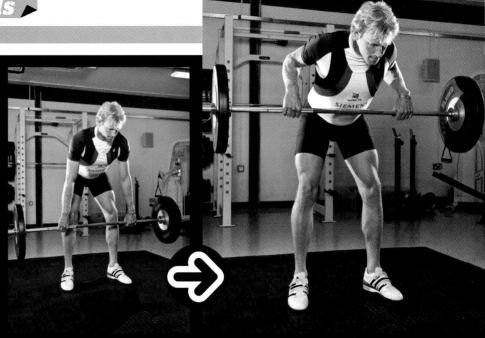

3 Bent-over row

Sets 3 **Reps** 6

> Lean forward at the hips and hold a bar at roughly knee height, keeping your back straight and neck in line with your spine. Brace your core and retract your shoulder blades as you pull the bar up to your sternum.

Hodge says
'The pull is the last part of the drive phase. It doesn't contribute so much to the speed of the boat, but if you lose control of the oar then you've lost control of the boat. You want your upper body to be strong and capable of handling what your legs can deliver.'

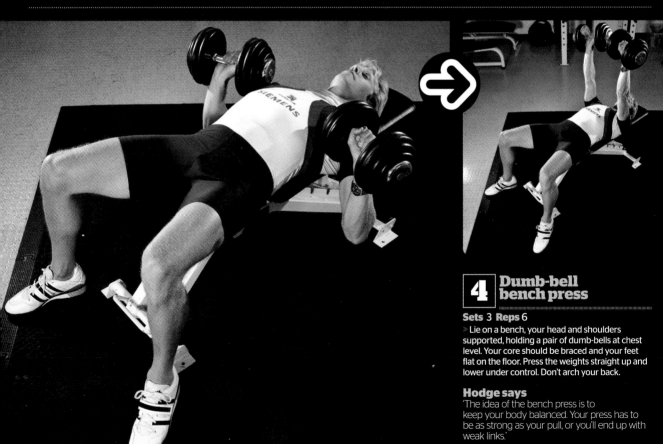

4 Dumb-bell bench press

Sets 3 **Reps** 6

> Lie on a bench, your head and shoulders supported, holding a pair of dumb-bells at chest level. Your core should be braced and your feet flat on the floor. Press the weights straight up and lower under control. Don't arch your back.

Hodge says
'The idea of the bench press is to keep your body balanced. Your press has to be as strong as your pull, or you'll end up with weak links.'

Part 2
CORE STRENGTH

'A huge amount of rowing is about holding a strong core,' says Hodge. 'So the exercises we do are about exposing the little muscles and engaging everything. A lot of it is neural, where you're trying to set up good working patterns. You don't want to just be good at rowing, you want to be good at a lot of things that contribute to good habits. Getting used to keeping a tight core is a big part

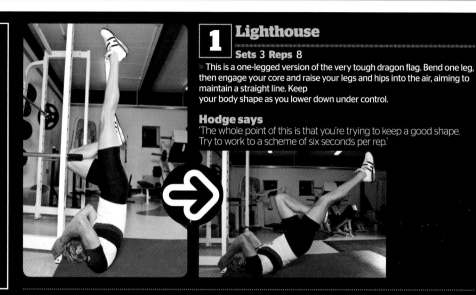

1 Lighthouse

Sets 3 **Reps** 8

This is a one-legged version of the very tough dragon flag. Bend one leg, then engage your core and raise your legs and hips into the air, aiming to maintain a straight line. Keep your body shape as you lower down under control.

Hodge says
'The whole point of this is that you're trying to keep a good shape. Try to work to a scheme of six seconds per rep.'

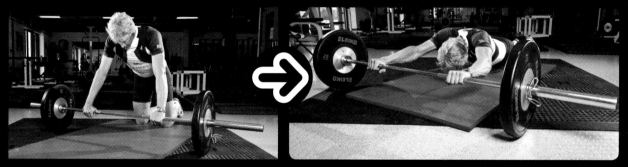

2 Barbell rollout

Sets 3 **Reps** 8

Get a barbell with big plates on either side. Kneel and hold the bar with your hands shoulder-width apart, then roll it forwards. If you can touch your chin to the ground, great, otherwise come back up when your hips start to sag.

Hodge says
'This'll take you through the full range of motion you'll go through during a rowing stroke and force you to keep tight all the time.'

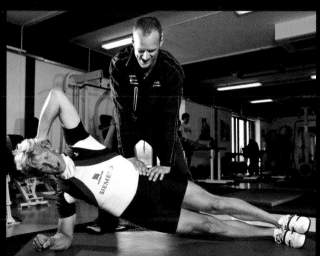

3 Resisted side plank

Sets 3 **Reps** 5 each side

You'll need a partner for this one. Get in a side plank with your forearm and bottom foot touching the floor, and get your partner to apply steady pressure downwards on your hip. Aim for an amount of pressure that will let you resist for around five seconds each rep.

Hodge says
'This is another move that develops the kind of unilateral core strength you need in the boat.'

GET SURF READY

Romain Cloître

Age 23
From Réunion
Achievements
■ 2007 Winner, ASP Junior European Tour
■ 2008 9th, Oakley Pro Junior Global Challenge
■ 2009 6th, European ASP World Qualifying Series

This workout from surf star Romain Cloître will improve your strength, power and stability and switch your muscles on before you paddle out

When you ride in one of the big international circuits, you'll be surfing different spots each week, and every new break will challenge you in different ways. 'This is why we need to do training above and beyond surfing,' says Cloître. 'Dry-land training helps us develop our natural attributes so we can perform at each event, no matter what the ocean throws at us.'

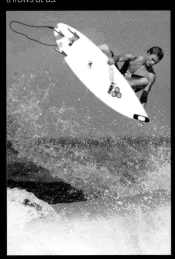

But finding the time or equipment to work out can be tricky when you're living out of a suitcase. 'I have a trainer, Fabien Uteau, who I work with five times a week when I'm in Réunion, but I can't bring him with me,' says Cloître. 'At a lot of the events I do my workouts on the beach, using a gym ball, medicine ball and a towel.

'On tour, I do four workouts a week, all of which are variations of the one you

'Dry land training helps us develop our natural attributes'

see here, aimed at developing my core stability, explosive power, strength and balance. The timing of the workouts is crucial – I do them as a morning warm-up just before I go in the sea because they activate all the muscles I'm going to use. This means I'm ready to surf as soon as I reach the ocean and I'm less likely to pull or strain anything because my tendons, ligaments and muscles are already warm and stretched. I do yoga-based stretching for 30 minutes when I get out to stay limber for the next session.' ⟩

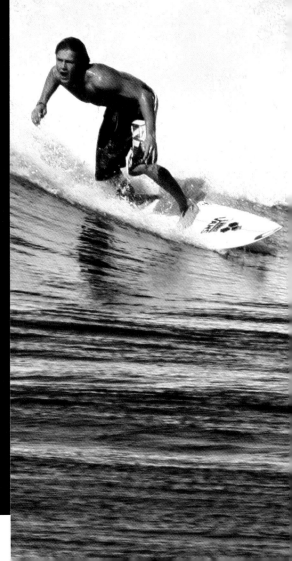

Part 1

UPPER-BODY STRENGTH AND EXPLOSIVE POWER

> 'By working your core, chest and arms at different tempos, these two exercises are excellent for improving your ability to paddle hard for long periods of time and pop up on your board in a quick, controlled way in unpredictable surf.'

1 Seal press-up

Sets 4 **Reps** 12

> Start with your arms just wider than shoulder-width apart and lean forward at the hips so your palms rest on the ground.

> Sink down, leading with your face. Your hips and legs should reach the lowest point of the move at the same time.

> As your hips reach the lowest position, push forward, then up with your head. Reverse the move to complete one rep.

Cloître says

'Even if I'm not doing a full workout, I always do this move as soon as I wake up – it's great for stretching and activating your entire body. Do it slowly so your muscles are under tension for longer.'

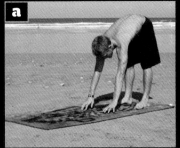
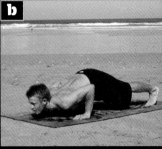
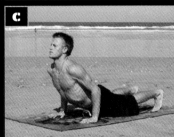
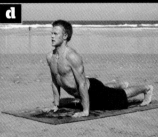

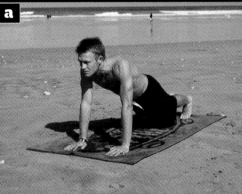
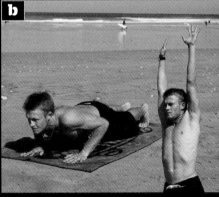
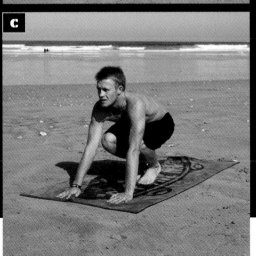
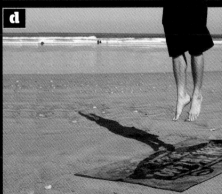

2 Press-up burpee

Sets 4 **Reps** 12

> Start in a press-up position with your arms shoulder-width apart.

> Sink down until your chest is about 15cm from the floor, keeping your body in a straight line and head facing forward.

> Press up and pull your legs forward explosively, carrying the explosion into a max effort vertical jump.

Cloître says

'The first half of this move mimics the pop-up technique you use to get into a standing position on your board. The jump helps you develop extra power, making what can be quite a demanding movement on the board feel effortless.'

Part 2
BALANCE AND LOWER-BODY STRENGTH

'Because a gym ball is an unstable platform and forces you to adopt a surf-style stance to stay steady, balancing on one will help you build surf-specific ankle strength and core stability,' says Cloître. 'The pay-off is that when you get into the water, this translates to better control of your turns and the ability to ride long, taxing waves without sacrificing form.'

1 Gym ball core rotation

Sets 4 **Reps** 20

> Start by inflating the gym ball to about 80 per cent of its capacity so it's easier to balance on. Inflate it more as you get used to doing the exercise.
> Adopt a crouched surf-like position on the ball and hold a light medicine ball out in front of you.
> Swing to the left then to the right, keeping your arms straight. That's one rep.

Cloître says
'When you start doing this joint-strengthening move, you might need a mate to help you get on to the ball and pass you the medicine ball. It also helps if you put the gym ball on a towel rather than sand, because the latter can be a bit slippery.'

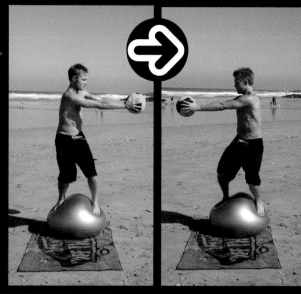

2 Gym ball squat

Sets 4 **Reps** 12

> Once you're on the ball, stand up as straight as you can. Hold your hands out in front of you for balance.
> Sink down slowly into as deep a squat as you can manage.

Cloître says
'I love this move because it works your lower body and core muscles the same way that surfing does – you're moving between the two stages of this exercise, albeit a bit faster when you're riding a wave.'

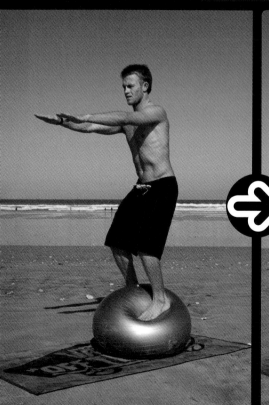

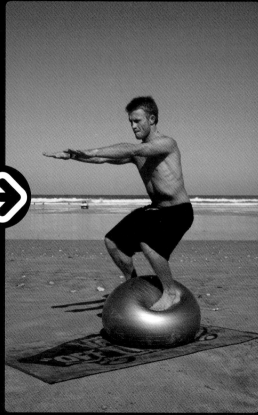

Part 3
CORE STABILITY

'Having a strong core helps you transfer upper-body power to your lower body so you can make powerful efficient movements on the board as well as helping you keep your balance,' says Cloître. 'Because you're constantly using your core during surfing, it will start to get tight when you're in the water for any serious amount of time, but the stabilising moves will keep the aches at bay for longer.'

1 Gym ball twisting sit-up

Sets 4 **Reps** 12 each side

➤ Sit on the ball, then lean back so your back wraps around it. Link your fingers behind your head.
➤ Contract your abs to lift your upper body off the ball.
➤ Curl to your left, bringing your hands out in front of you so you touch your left foot at the bottom of the move.

Cloître says:
'Surfing is such a twisty sport so you need to strengthen the muscles – your obliques and underlying chest muscles – that transfer turning power from your upper to your lower body.'

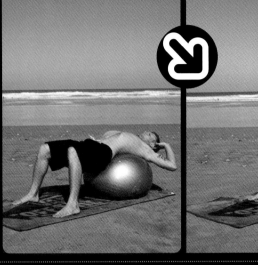
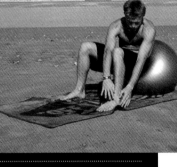

2 Two-point box

Sets 4 **Reps** 12 each side

➤ Kneel on all fours with your head facing forward and your back straight.
➤ Kick your right leg out and stretch out your left hand as far as you can. Hold the position for a two-count.
➤ Repeat to the other side, keeping your abdominals braced throughout each rep.

Cloître says:
'The quick, forceful movements you make while surfing can jar your back, but by stabilising and strengthening the muscles around your spine, this simple move will protect this injury-prone area.'

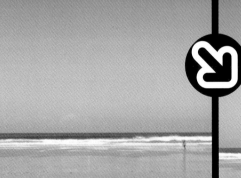
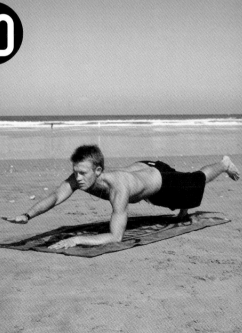

Photography **Sam Mellish, Laurent Capmas**

TRI TRAIN LIKE A CHAMPION

Triathlete Will Clarke on racing hard and mid-race mental toughness

How is training going?
I'm feeling better than ever. I've cut out the mad weeks – I used to be a big trainer but I found if I did 35 hours one week, I'd do 28 the next then 15 after that because I was so knackered. Now I'm more consistent. I've only gone over 30 hours a week a couple of times this year.

How mentally tough is racing?
It screws with your mind. Everyone is trying to attack you and everyone is hurting as much as each other. It's about who wants it most.

What's the hardest part?
The last 3km of a run is when it gets very tough and everyone is starting to think seriously about the win.

How is the competition among the British triathletes at the moment?
It's very good. To be honest, it's too good! We've got the Brownlee brothers, Alistair and Jonathan. Alistair is extremely hard to beat and everyone's scratching their heads wondering how he's doing it.

Can you beat him?
I hope so. I think the only way to do it is to run faster and be the strongest at the end of the race.

What is your Olympic goal?
Everyone is going for a medal, including me. Preferably, it'll be a gold.

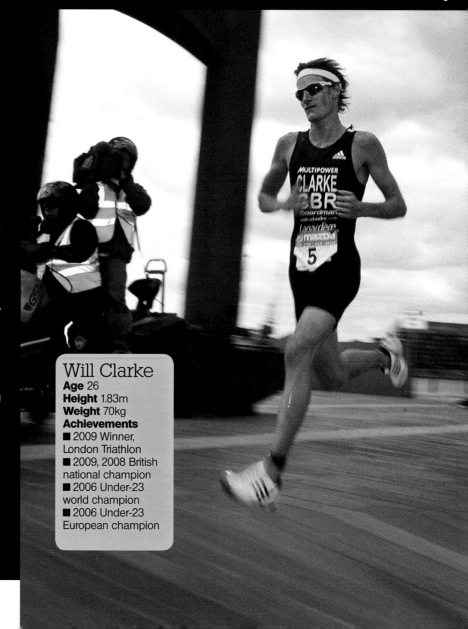

Will Clarke
Age 26
Height 1.83m
Weight 70kg
Achievements
■ 2009 Winner, London Triathlon
■ 2009, 2008 British national champion
■ 2006 Under-23 world champion
■ 2006 Under-23 European champion

Part 1
CORE STRENGTH

'Good posture and core strength is imperative for a triathlete – especially in the switch from cycling, where the spine is flexed, to running, where you aim to remain upright and extended in order to run efficiently,' says Clarke's strength and conditioning coach, Mark Niemz, who's employed by the English Institute of Sport to train Britain's Olympic triathlon squad. 'Good core stability during swimming allows the athlete to remain in a streamlined position and catch the water [push water behind you and propel yourself forward] during the stroke. This will connect what you do with your arms to your trunk and hips, allowing you to use your whole body to drive your arm propulsion, and not overwork the shoulder and upper back muscles.'

TRX trainer complex

Sets 3 Do 1a, 1b and 1c back to back without rest.

Clarke's tip
The TRX trainer is a convenient way to do core endurance sets because you hold the fixed trunk position, working your shoulders and core, while moving at the knee and hip.'

1a Pike
Reps 15

> Get into a press-up position with your feet in the handles of the TRX trainer a few centimetres off the floor. Contract your abs to raise your backside up, making your body into an inverted V.

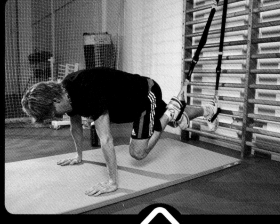

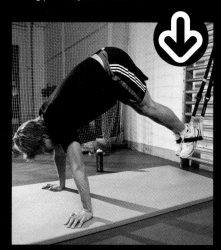

1b Running
Reps 15

> Get into a press-up position with your feet in the handles of the TRX trainer a few centimetres off the floor. Bring one knee in towards your chest then, as you return it to the start position, bring your other knee in towards your chest.

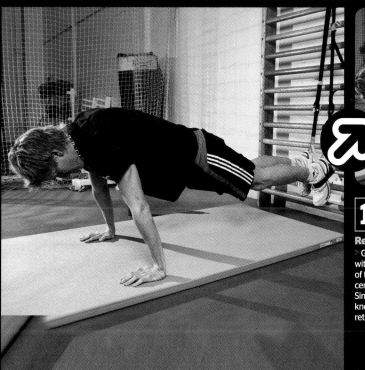

1c Knee tuck
Reps 15

> Get into a press-up position with your feet in the handles of the TRX trainer a few centimetres off the floor. Simultaneously bring both knees in to your chest then return to the start position.

Part 2
GLUTE AND HAMSTRING STRENGTH

'This is important for running. It focuses on the muscles of the posterior chain – the ones down the back of your body,' says Niemz. 'It's an area that athletes can be weak in, particularly if they do a lot of cycling, which makes them disproportionately strong in the quads and hip flexors. During a triathlon you spend an hour on the bike, doing thousands of pedal strokes in a flexed-hip position. You go from that to an upright position for the run, which requires glute and

1 Weighted glute bridge

Sets 3 **Reps** 10-15

▷ Lie with your back on the floor, your knees bent and a barbell across your hips. Contract your glutes and raise your hips off the floor.

Clarke says
'If you find it difficult to go low during squats (below the point where your thighs are parallel to the floor), which is when your glutes and hamstrings are recruited most, this is a good alternate way of overloading the glutes.'

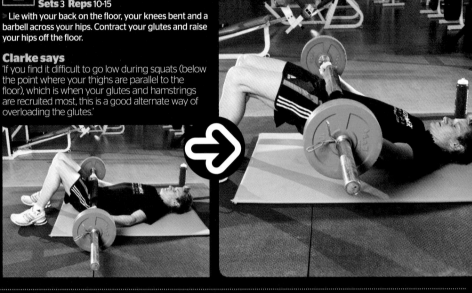

2 Split squat

Sets 3-4 **Reps** 6-10 each side

▷ Start in a split stance with your body upright and a barbell across your back. Keeping your core braced and your back upright, lower until both your front and back knees are bent at 90˚.

Clarke says
'Doing a split squat rather than a conventional squat makes it more cycling-specific. It's an easy way to go deep with a flexed hip and knee and will help improve your power output on the bike.'

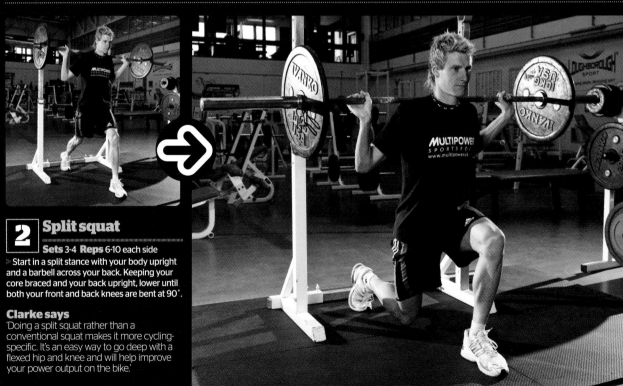

Part 3
UPPER-BODY STRENGTH

'You need good upper-body strength in the swim so we work on both vertical and horizontal pulling movements,' says Niemz. 'We use generic upper-body moves such as the chin-up to strengthen the back and swimming-specific moves

1 TRX inverted row

Sets 3 **Reps** 8-10
▶ Hold the TRX trainer with your arms straight and your body in a straight line off the floor. Raise your body by rowing the TRX trainer to your chest.

Clarke says
'We do this on a TRX rather than a bar because it allows you to externally rotate the shoulders. You start with your palms facing down and rotate your arms so your palms face inwards at the top of the move.'

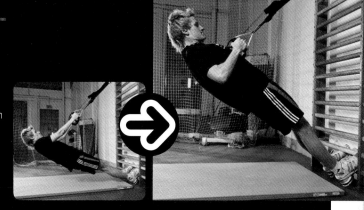

2 Dumb-bell pullover

Sets 3 **Reps** 10-15
▶ Lie on a bench holding a dumb-bell behind your head, arms straight. Keeping them straight, raise the dumb-bell until it is above your chest.

Clarke says
This is more specific to the swimming stroke than a pull-up.'

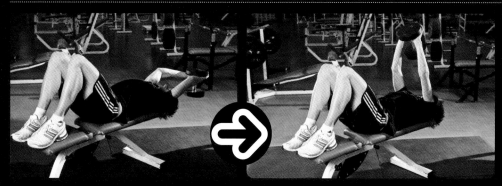

3 Pull-up complex

▶ Do one set to failure of the following pull-up variations
3a Wide-grip
Take a wide grip and pull up until your chin is over the bar.
3b Hammer-grip
With palms facing each other, pull up until your chin is over the bar.
3c Chin-up
Use an underhand grip and pull up until your chin is over the bar.

Clarke says
'Variations on a move let you do more reps than if you did just one movement. We concentrate on the wide grip because it activates the lats, making it more swimming-specific.'

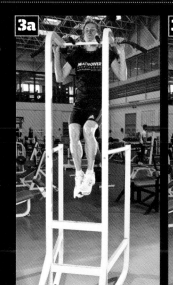

3a

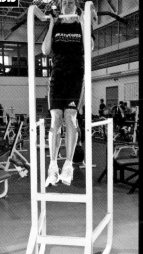

3b

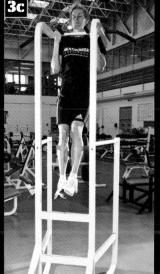

3c

Photography **Tom Miles** Will Clarke is an ambassador for Multipower sports nutrition. Visit multipoweruk.com

CLIMB EVERY MOUNTAIN

Fearless British climber Leo Houlding has tackled challenges from El Capitan in California to Everest. Here's how he prepares himself in the gym

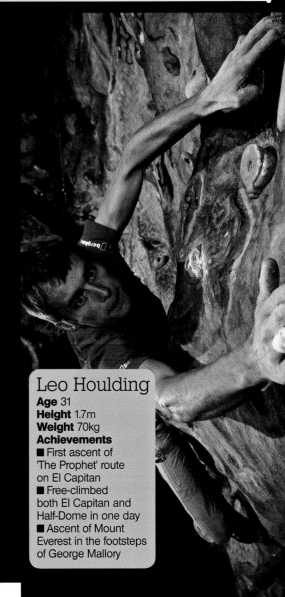

Last year you nailed the Prophet. Just how tough was it?

I've been trying the route for nine years, I've spent more than 60 days on that piece of the rock. When we did the free ascent it took six days, but four of those were spent in a godawful storm. So there were only two climbing days. We sat on a portaledge that flooded in full storm conditions, for more than 80 hours without moving, in a 4ft by 6ft tent, completely soaked and cold, borderline hypothermic, and then we had to dry everything out for a day and a half and go and perform at our absolute peak.

What was the hardest part in terms of climbing technique?

The really difficult bit is this feature called the A1 Beauty: it's a beautiful, 35m crack up a totally flat wall. There's nothing for your hands, nothing for your feet – just this minute crack to jam your fingertips in. And at that point you're more than twice as high as Canary Wharf.

Do you train on indoor walls?

Well, I'm a professional so I get to chase the summer around the world, which means I tend not to train inside that

> **'A base level of fitness is important. I tend to get out on my mountain bike'**

much. But if you live in the city, in the winter it's not easy to train in the field. There's a lot of crossover between styles of climbing, so if you want to do big wall climbing you can get some of the benefits by training indoors. Even on a high cliff it comes down to the individual moves, which you can do by bouldering.

What's a typical training session on a wall like for you?

If I'm on a lead wall [one on which you clip your rope in as you ascend], the classic thing I do to train for endurance on the big cliffs is start on a route that's graded relatively easy for me like a 6a, then do a 6a-plus, then a 6b, then go all the way up to an 8a-plus, then I'm usually pretty tired so I might fall off that, then I'll go all the way up and back down. That's about 28 pitches if you go all the way up and back down again, which should take a couple of hours.

Do pull-ups help your climbing?

Although you need a basic level of strength, I wouldn't recommend loads of pull-ups, especially if you're a beginner. It's much more important to focus on technique. One of the reasons women often make good climbers is that they usually don't have that upper-body strength, so they have to focus on technique. Also, a base level of fitness is important, so you can go on the cross-trainer or on a bike. I tend to get out on my mountain bike for fitness. >

Leo Houlding
Age 31
Height 1.7m
Weight 70kg
Achievements
■ First ascent of 'The Prophet' route on El Capitan
■ Free-climbed both El Capitan and Half-Dome in one day
■ Ascent of Mount Everest in the footsteps of George Mallory

Part 1
CLIMBING STRENGTH

> 'The best training for climbing is climbing,' says Houlding. 'Men who come from a gym background tend to think they can do everything by pulling. But someone with good technique will definitely outperform someone with loads of strength but bad technique.'

1 Circuit training

'If you don't have access to a roped climbing wall or a partner, circuits are the best way to make the most of a bouldering wall,' says Houlding. 'You can do a circuit by yourself, and it only takes an hour or two to have a really good session. Find a circuit that requires about 70 per cent of your ability, not too difficult or too easy, containing anything between 35 and 65 separate moves. Ideally you don't want moves that go sideways – in real rock climbing you won't go sideways that much. Do the circuit, have two or three minutes' rest, then go again. You might only be able to do it a few times at first. When you can do it without getting tired, add in some harder moves.'

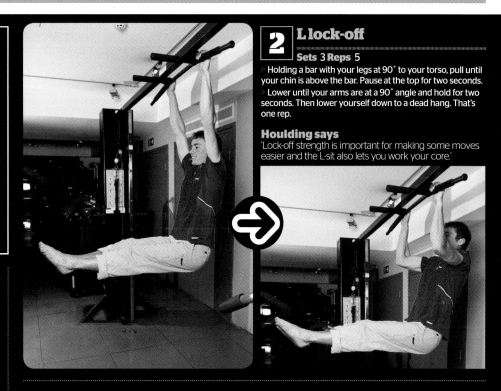

2 L lock-off
Sets 3 Reps 5

> Holding a bar with your legs at 90° to your torso, pull until your chin is above the bar. Pause at the top for two seconds.
> Lower until your arms are at a 90° angle and hold for two seconds. Then lower yourself down to a dead hang. That's one rep.

Houlding says
'Lock-off strength is important for making some moves easier and the L-sit also lets you work your core.'

3 Around the world
Sets 3 Reps 5

> Grab a pull-up bar with an overhand grip. Pull up to your left so your head ends up close to your left arm. Pull yourself across to the right, and lower from there.

> Repeat but pull up to the right and lower from the left. That's one rep.

Houlding says
'This works your shoulders at angles a pull-up won't hit.'

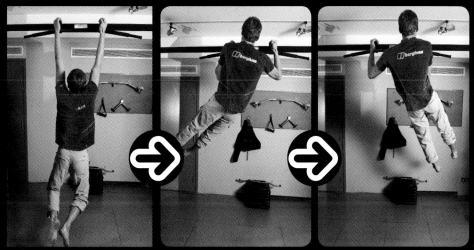

Part 2
CORE STRENGTH

'Even when you're overhanging, climbing is still about keeping your weight over your feet,' says Houlding. 'That's where your core comes in. You need a really strong core just to be able to keep your feet on the wall.'

1 Plank leg raise

Sets 2
Reps 5 each side
> Hold yourself in a plank, keeping your body in a straight line from your shoulders to your feet.
> Raise one foot and hold it for two seconds before lowering. Repeat on the other side.

Houlding says
'You shouldn't let your hips move at all during this move. If it's too easy, you're probably shifting to one side.'

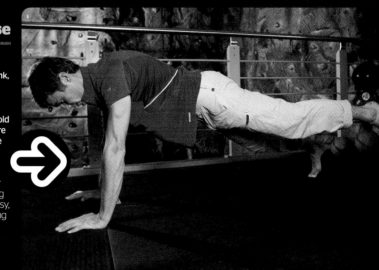

2 Side plank cross

Sets 2 **Reps** 5 each side
> Hold yourself in a side plank, with one foot on the floor, your body straight and one arm raised.
> Raise your top leg until it's at a roughly 45° angle with your bottom leg.
> Hold for two seconds, then lower it.

Houlding says
'I do this a lot, with some other Pilates moves that I can do pretty much wherever I am.'

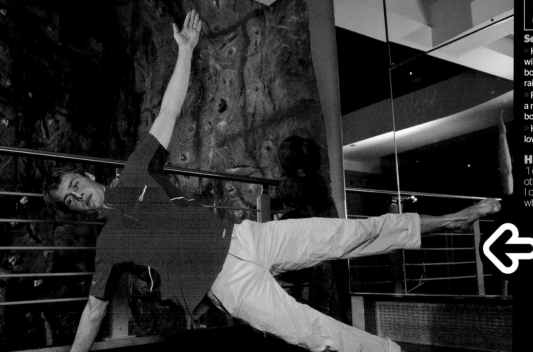

'I blew my medial collateral ligament last year so now I do a lot of stability work as rehab, but also as prehab, to stop me doing it again,' says Houlding. 'A lot of it's based around balance and proprioception [teaching the body about movement patterns]. Do it on a wobble cushion or a Bosu rather than a wobble board.'

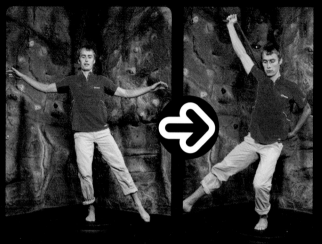

1 One-legged balance

> Stand on a Bosu or wobble cushion on one leg.
> Perform a half-squat, making sure your knee tracks forward over your second toe. Hold it for 20 seconds, then straighten back up, keeping the move controlled throughout.

Houlding says
'You're supposed to be wobbling during this move. If you aren't, it won't work your proprioception properly.'

Harder variation

2 Bosu balance stretch

> Stand on one leg on a Bosu and hold a stretch band behind your back as you stretch it.
> When you feel the stretch, hold for 30 seconds.
> For a harder variation, loop the band around one foot and use it to stretch your leg.

Houlding says
'The stretching element will help you with your mobility, but it's also to make balancing harder.'

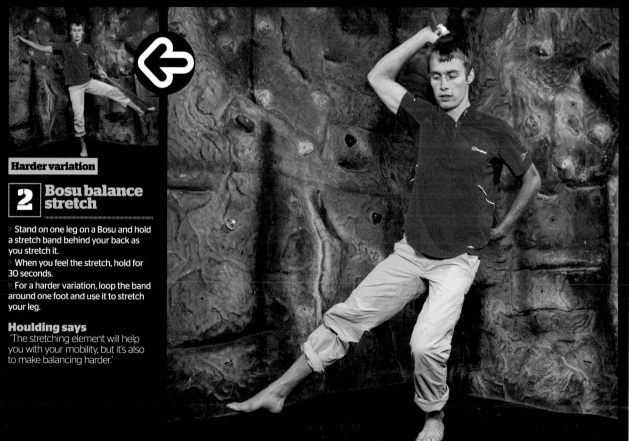

Photography Tom Miles

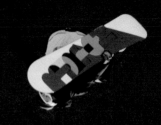

ABOVE BOARD

Veteran Slovenian freestyle snowboarder Marko Grilc takes *MF* through the exercises that prepare him for pulling big tricks

At 28, you're one of freestyle snowboarding's older pros. How has age affected the way you ride and train?
I have to do way more off-board training to stay at the forefront of the sport than I did when I was younger. In the off-season I run four times a week, normally for more than an hour – this gives me the endurance I need to keep pulling big tricks all day. I also work with a personal trainer in Croatia to improve my balance and build my leg strength. The gym is definitely an old snowboarder's best friend.

So you've become more disciplined as you've got older?
Yeah, I've come a long way from just partying every day and throwing myself off cliffs. But going for it fully is what snowboarding should always be about.

How soon into a training session do you start doing difficult tricks, such as double flips and massive spins?
If I'm feeling really good, I'll start trying difficult technical tricks immediately. But normally I'll do a lesser rotation during my first jump then go for something bigger off the second kicker.

How much attention do you pay to your diet?
I used to eat whatever I wanted to but now I try to be healthier. If I'm snowboarding in a park, I normally go to a restaurant for a well-balanced lunch rather than carry food up the hill. If I'm riding backcountry, I carry a litre of water to keep me hydrated and things to give me a quick hit of energy, such as fruit and chocolate.

You won London Freeze in 2010 after dislocating your hip during the 2009 event. Did that mean a lot to you?
I had to really battle to perform there because the 2009 fall was always at the back of my mind. Winning really helped me overcome my hang-ups about my hip, which felt like more of an achievement than getting a medal. It had taken me about three months to recover physically from the fall but mentally, the damage lasts much longer. It forces you to realise how easily one bad slam could end your career.

How often do you scare yourself when you're riding?
All the time. In an environment as competitive as snowboarding you get left behind if you stay in your comfort zone.

> 'The gym is definitely an old snowboarder's best friend'

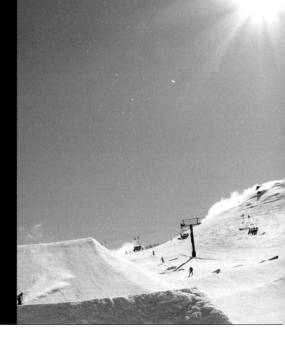

Part 1
LEG AND BACK MOBILITY

'Your legs and feet are the parts of your body that have to work the hardest during any trick,' says Grilc. 'You rely on them to spring into the air and they have to soak up the impact when you land, so you need them to be strong and flexible.'

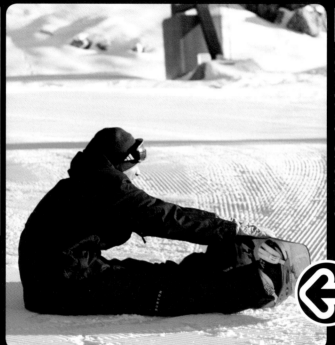

1 Sitting reach
Sets 3 **Time** 20 seconds
> Strap on your snowboard and sit down on the floor with a slight bend in your knees.
> Reach forward and grab the front edge of your snowboard between your legs with both hands.
> Straighten your legs as far as is comfortable and hold.

Grilc says
'As well as your hamstrings and calves, this also stretches your back and arms, which is crucial because it's easy to pull or strain something if you start busting out spins with cold muscles.'

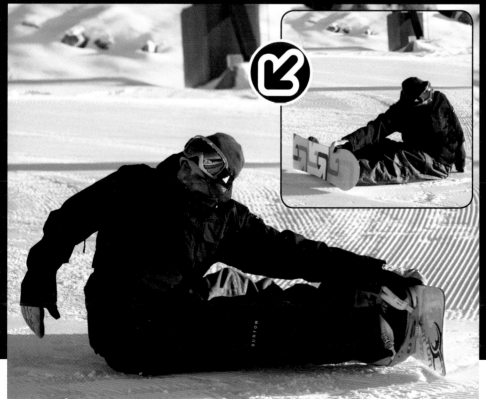

2 Grab stretch
Sets 2 **Time** 20 seconds each side
> Sit with your legs as straight as you can and grab the front edge of the board with one hand.
> Twist your torso away from your grabbing hand and use your other hand to stop you toppling over if you need to.

Grilc says
'This puts your body under the same kind of tension and positions it'll be in when you pull tricks off kickers. I do this as soon as I get out of the gondola, so my muscles are fully activated before I start riding.'

Part 2
CORE STRENGTH AND FLEXIBILITY

> 'A strong midsection is essential,' says Grilc. 'Your core transfers movement from your upper to your lower body when you spin, enabling you to complete rotations. It also stabilises you when you land and improves your balance and posture for backcountry hikes through deep snow.'

1 Core rotation

Sets 3 **Reps** 10 each side

> Stand with your feet just wider than shoulder-width apart holding your board against your lower back with the bindings facing away from you.
> Make sure the nose of the board is sticking out further than the tail.
> Rotate your upper body as far as you can one way, then the other. That's one rep.
> Keep your feet anchored in place throughout the move
> Once you've done ten reps, shuffle the board along so the tail is sticking out further than the nose and repeat the reps.

Grilc says
'This move mimics the twist your torso goes through during a spin. Having more weight on one side brings your obliques into play to keep your feet rooted to the spot.'

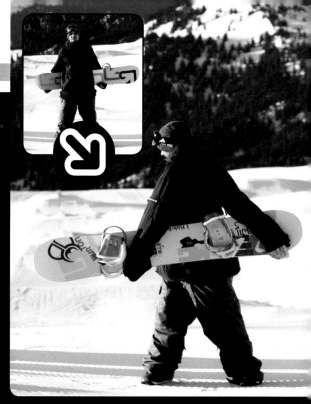

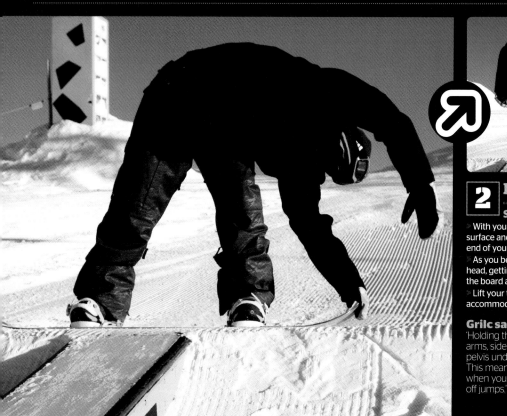

2 Exaggerated grab

Sets 2 **Time** 20 seconds each side

> With your board strapped on, stand on a flat surface and lean over to one side, grabbing the end of your board with your leading hand.
> As you bend, bring your other hand over your head, getting it as close as you can to the end of the board and hold.
> Lift your trailing leg and twist your hips to accommodate the movement.

Grilc says
'Holding this exaggerated pose puts your back, arms, side abs and the muscles around your pelvis under more strain than doing tricks will. This means your body will feel comfortable when you start throwing nose and tail grabs off jumps.'

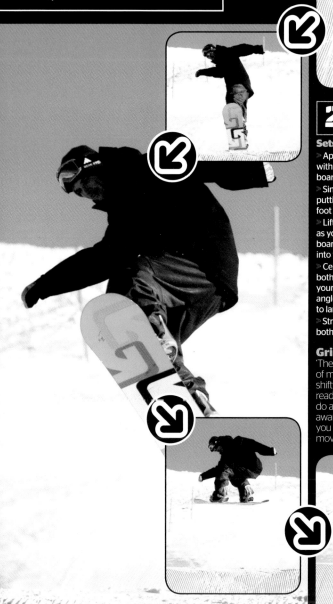

Part 3
EXPLOSIVE POWER

> 'As well as the stamina to keep riding all day during a competition, a pro rider needs bags of explosive power because you're going to be constantly popping on to, over and off obstacles,' says Grilc.

1 Board presses

Sets 3 **Reps** 10 each side

> With your board strapped on, stand on a flat surface.

> Bring one end of the board off the ground by leaning towards the other end. As you reach the outer limit of your balance, use the board's spring to flick you back the other way.

> Land with your weight over your other foot, so the previously grounded side of the board is off the floor, then lean over until you've generated enough recoil to spring yourself back the other way.

Grilc says

'You want to do this fast to mimic the plyometric effect of pulling combo tricks on rails and boxes. If you jump forward slightly during each rep, it also becomes an effective way of moving up mellow hills without having to unstrap.'

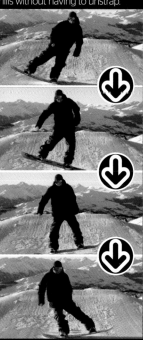

2 Shifty ollie

Sets 1 **Reps** 5 each side

> Approach a small jump or bump with your weight centred over the board.

> Sink down as you reach the lip, putting your weight over your back foot to spring-load the board.

> Lift your front foot off the ground as you lean back, then use the board's spring to get your back foot into the air too.

> Centre your weight as you get both feet into the air, then twist your hips to one side so the board is angled away from where you want to land.

> Straighten the board and land on both feet at the same time.

Grilc says

'The ollie or jump is the essence of most snowboard tricks. The shifty gets your hips and core ready for all the twisting they'll do and increases your spatial awareness in the air, preparing you for bigger, more technical moves.'

Photography Cyril Müller

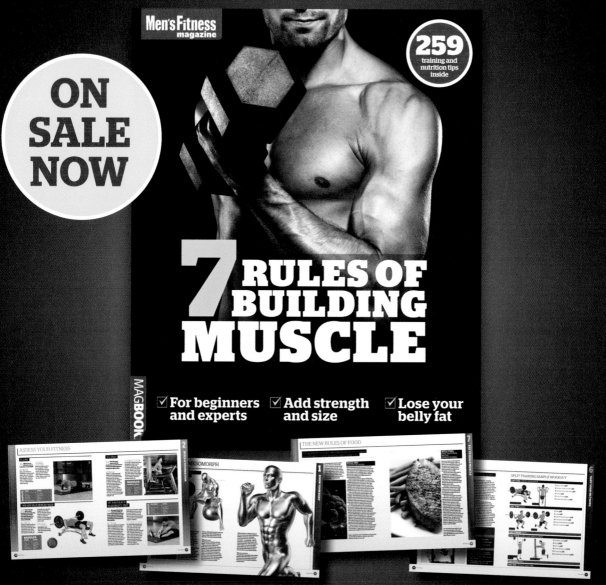

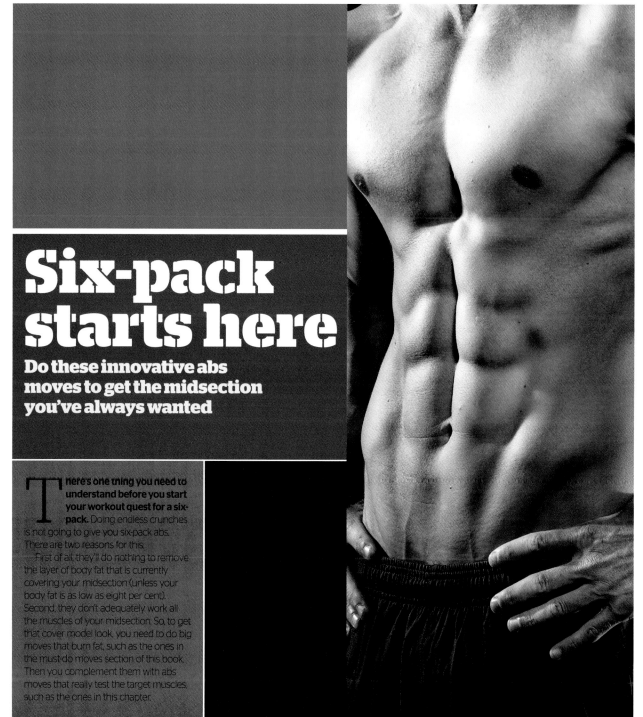

Six-pack starts here

Do these innovative abs moves to get the midsection you've always wanted

There's one thing you need to understand before you start your workout quest for a six-pack. Doing endless crunches is not going to give you six-pack abs. There are two reasons for this.

First of all, they'll do nothing to remove the layer of body fat that is currently covering your midsection (unless your body fat is as low as eight per cent). Second, they don't adequately work all the muscles of your midsection. So, to get that cover model look, you need to do big moves that burn fat, such as the ones in the must-do moves section of this book. Then you complement them with abs moves that really test the target muscles, such as the ones in this chapter.

Vertical twist

Sets 4
Reps 10

Blast your abs from top to bottom and hit your internal obliques as well

STAGE 1

> Lie on your back with your feet together and your legs straight up in the air.

> Raise your hips off the ground and twist to the right until your legs are at 45° to the floor. Make sure you lower slowly and under control, using your muscles to control the move rather than letting gravity do the work.

> Return to the top of the move and repeat to the left. Alternate with each rep.

STAGE 2

STAGE 3

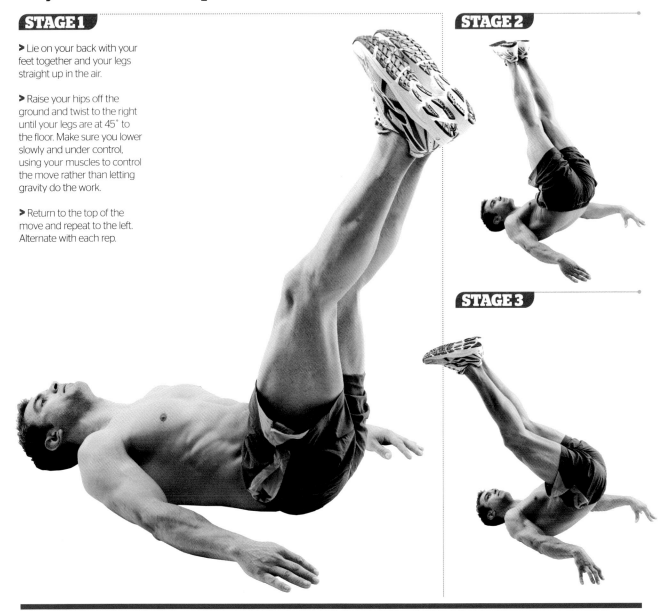

Plank walkout

Turn the humble plank into a dynamic test of abdominal strength and core stability

Sets 3
Reps 15

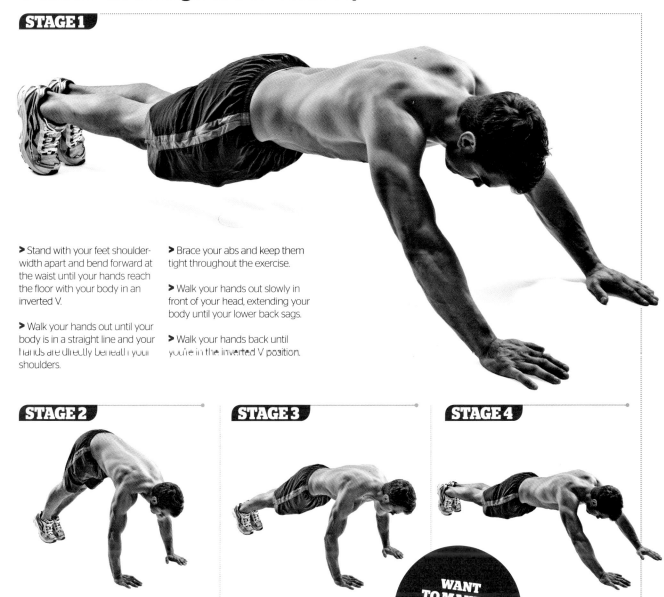

> Stand with your feet shoulder-width apart and bend forward at the waist until your hands reach the floor with your body in an inverted V.

> Walk your hands out until your body is in a straight line and your hands are directly beneath your shoulders.

> Brace your abs and keep them tight throughout the exercise.

> Walk your hands out slowly in front of your head, extending your body until your lower back sags.

> Walk your hands back until you're in the inverted V position.

STAGE 2

STAGE 3

STAGE 4

WANT TO MAKE IT HARDER?
Raise one leg

Ball side plank

Hit your abs from the side to build a solid six-pack

Sets 3
Reps 10 each side

STAGE 1

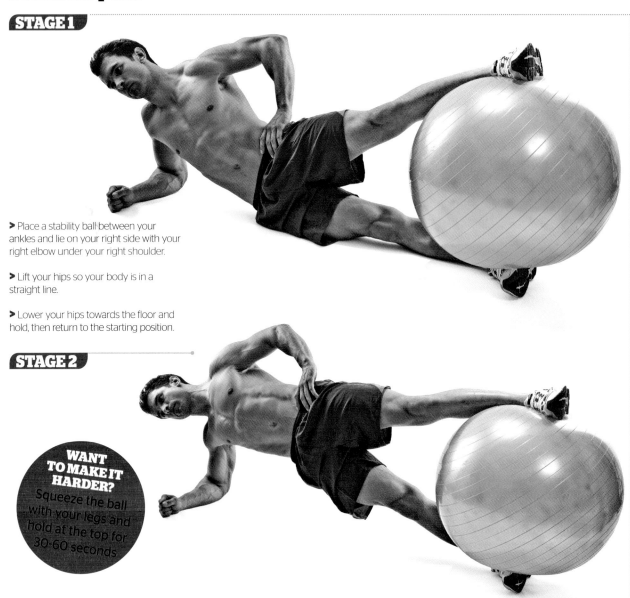

> Place a stability ball between your ankles and lie on your right side with your right elbow under your right shoulder.

> Lift your hips so your body is in a straight line.

> Lower your hips towards the floor and hold, then return to the starting position.

STAGE 2

WANT TO MAKE IT HARDER? Squeeze the ball with your legs and hold at the top for 30-60 seconds

Mountain climber

Sets 4
Time 45 seconds

Target the entire core and improve your muscular endurance

STAGE 1

> Get in a plank position with your hands on either side of a Bosu (round side down) and your body in a straight line from head to toe.

> Tighten your abs, then drive one knee up to your elbows.

> Alternate sides.

STAGE 2

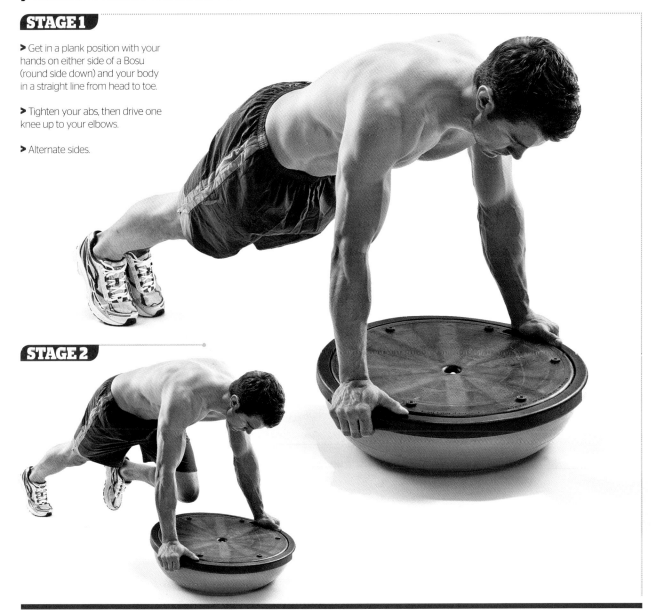

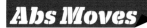

Jackknife twist

Sets 3
Reps 10

**Challenge your core and build strong abs
while working your shoulders and lower back**

STAGE 1

STAGE 2

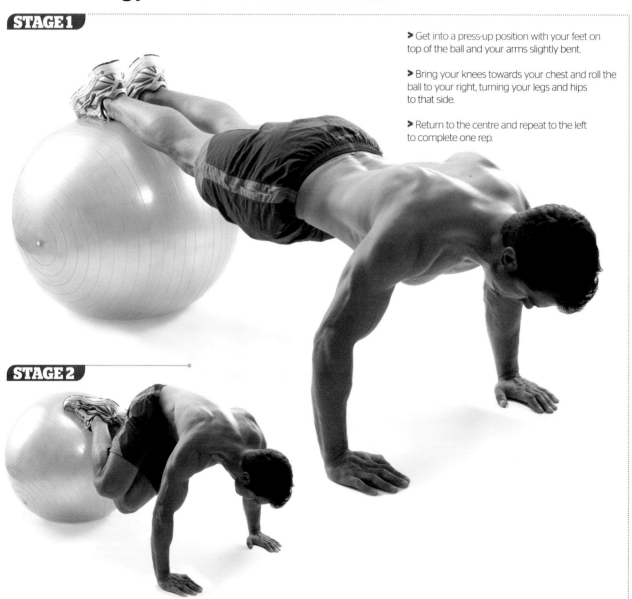

> Get into a press-up position with your feet on top of the ball and your arms slightly bent.

> Bring your knees towards your chest and roll the ball to your right, turning your legs and hips to that side.

> Return to the centre and repeat to the left to complete one rep.

Band sit-up

Work your core and chest with a Bosu ball and resistance band

Sets 3
Time 12-15

STAGE 1

> Sit on a Bosu ball with a resistance band secured behind you, your knees bent and your feet flat on the floor.

> Hold the handle slightly above your chest, palms facing forward, and raise your head and shoulders.

> Sit up as you straighten your arms, pushing the handle away from you. Pause, then lower to the starting position and repeat.

STAGE 2

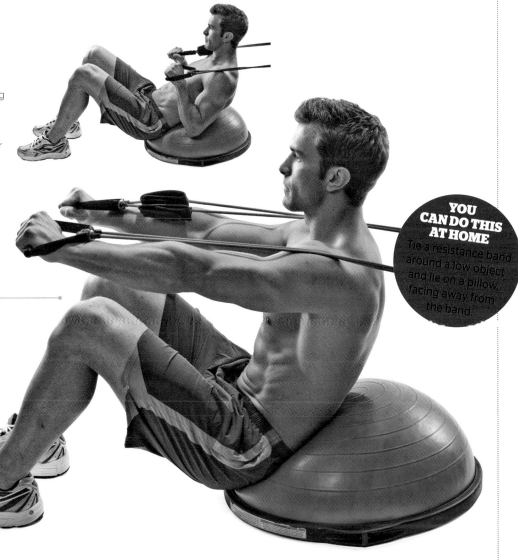

YOU CAN DO THIS AT HOME
Tie a resistance band around a low object and lie on a pillow, facing away from the band.

Side plank touch

Give the side plank a twist for an extra abs challenge

Sets 3
Reps 12-15

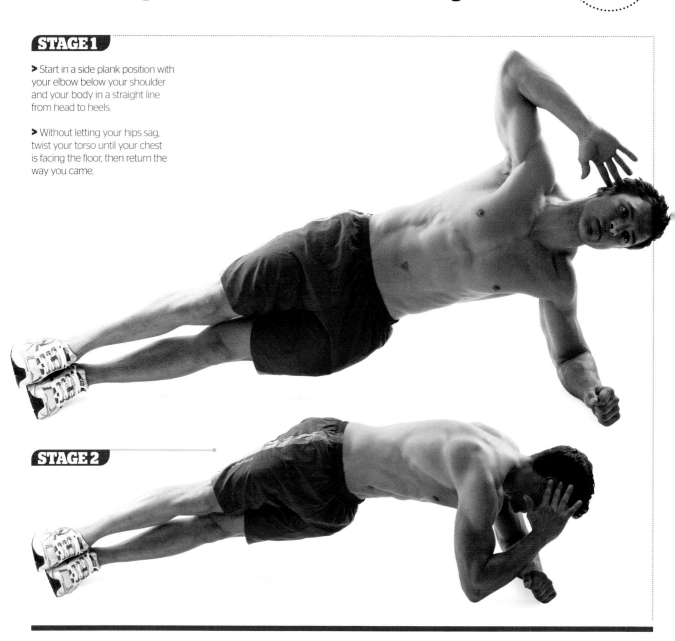

STAGE 1

> Start in a side plank position with your elbow below your shoulder and your body in a straight line from head to heels.

> Without letting your hips sag, twist your torso until your chest is facing the floor, then return the way you came.

STAGE 2

Pole push

Get hard abs while also building your core and lower back

Sets 3
Reps 12

STAGE 1

> Kneel on the floor, holding a metre-long pole with your arms outstretched at shoulder height.

> Make sure the pole is planted in the ground about a metre in front of your hands.

> Move the pole into an upright position by contracting your abs and extending your body straight from hands to hips.

> Make sure your back doesn't hyperextend and return slowly to the start.

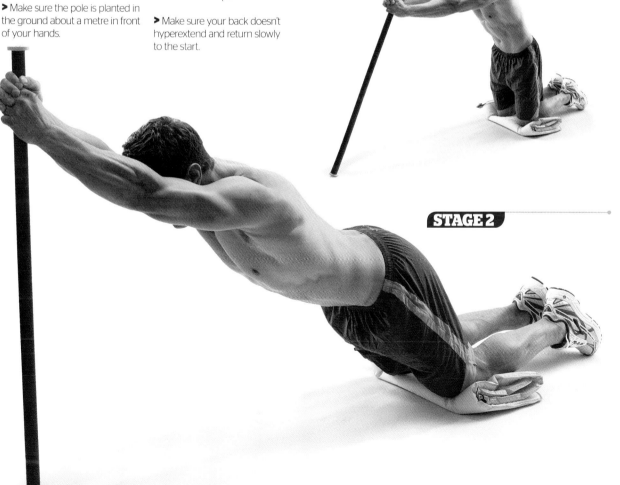

STAGE 2

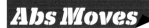
Side plank snatch

Sets 4
Reps 12

Add an extra hit to the side plank to strengthen your abs, back and hips

STAGE 1

> Start in the bottom position of a side plank with one arm straight and your hip on the floor.

> Grab a dumb-bell or kettlebell (start relatively light to assess your strength) and lift the weight above your body in a straight line with your free arm, using a snatch motion.

> Lower the weight back down before performing the move again.

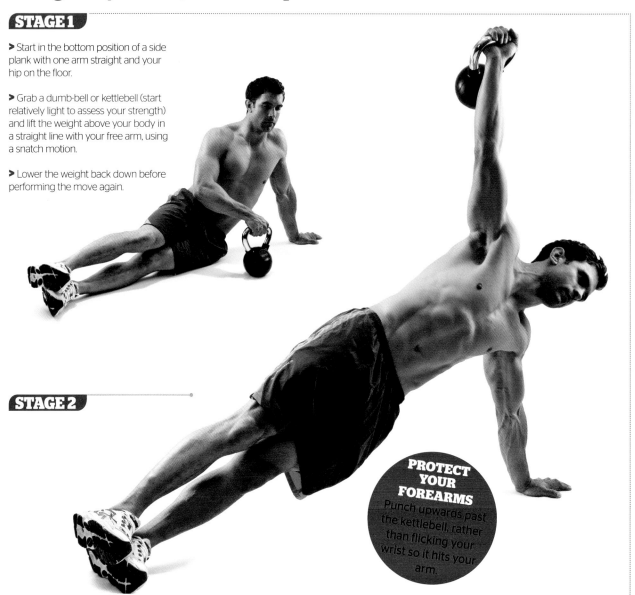

STAGE 2

PROTECT YOUR FOREARMS
Punch upwards past the kettlebell, rather than flicking your wrist so it hits your arm.

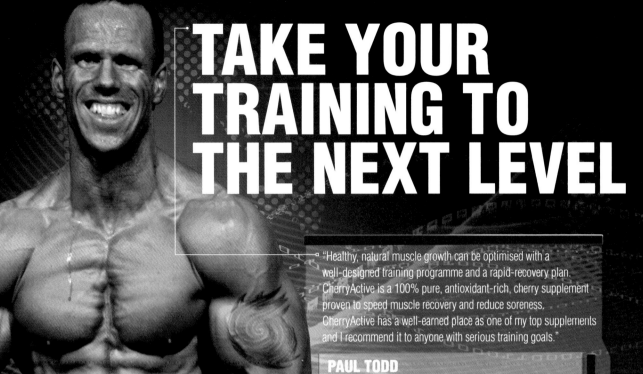
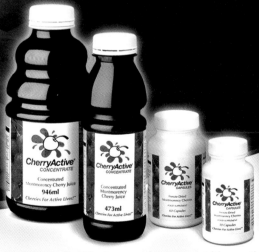

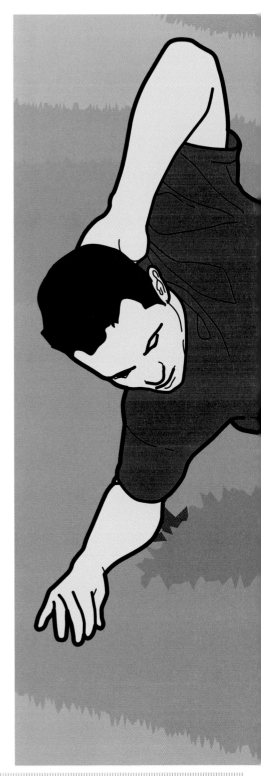

Fat loss furnace

Do these circuits to blast away your belly

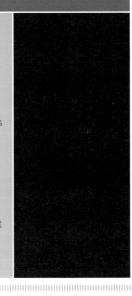

A lot of people mistakenly think that the best way to lose fat is to embark on long, slow runs. In fact, the most effective way of getting rid of your spare tyre is to do resistance exercise circuits.

Studies have shown that resistance training will burn more calories than steady-state cardio because your body burns lots of calories during the session and also afterwards as it recovers. An added benefit is that resistance training helps to build muscle, which is active tissue that, unlike fat, helps to burn even more calories. So by building muscle you are also helping yourself to lose fat.

Arranging your workouts in a circuit, where you take minimal rest between exercises, helps to keep your heart rate up so you're working hard throughout the session. The benefit of this is that the sessions are relatively short – about half an hour. To keep things interesting we've themed each one so you've got an arsenal of sessions to use in your fat attack. Your belly fat doesn't stand a chance.

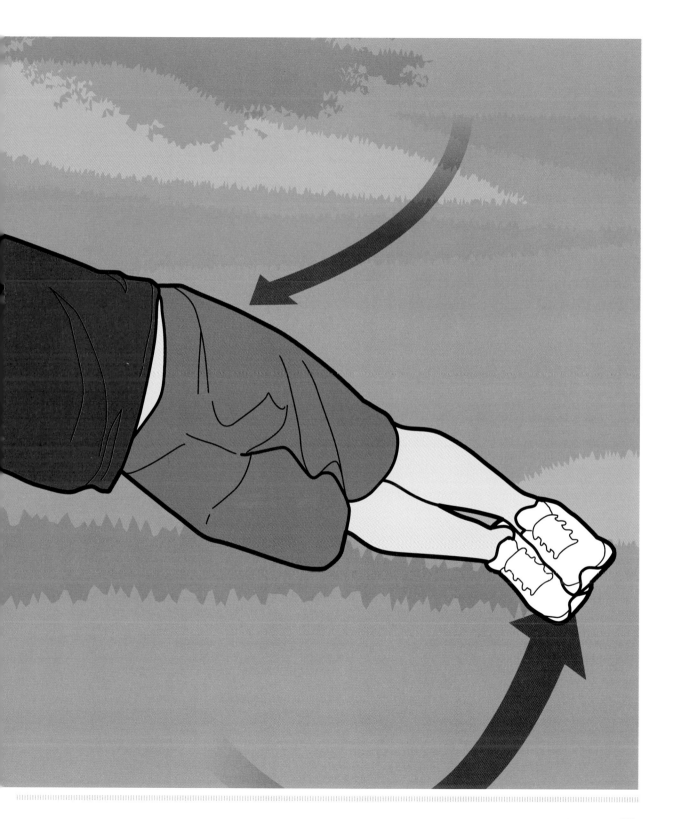

Blast your abs

See off the fat and build abs to be proud of with this killer circuit

How it works ▸

To get an impressive six-pack you need not only to build your abs but also to get rid of the layer of fat that covers them. This circuit has both parts covered – it hits all the muscles in the abdominal wall and burns serious amounts of calories.

You start with exercises that switch on your core's stabilising muscles so your stomach muscles are completed warmed up and ready to work to their full potential. The moves then get progressively harder, hitting the abs from different angles and raising your heart rate. The stabilising moves will help protect your back during this harder section.

Do all the exercises in order, with 30 seconds of medicine ball abs slams after each move to activate fast-twitch muscles and burn loads of fat. Complete the circuit twice.

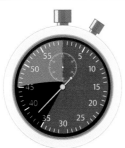

Time per session
35 minutes

Calorie burn
350

Illustrations **Stuart Holmes@Illustrationweb** The amount of calories burned will vary depending on your bodyweight and ×thess level

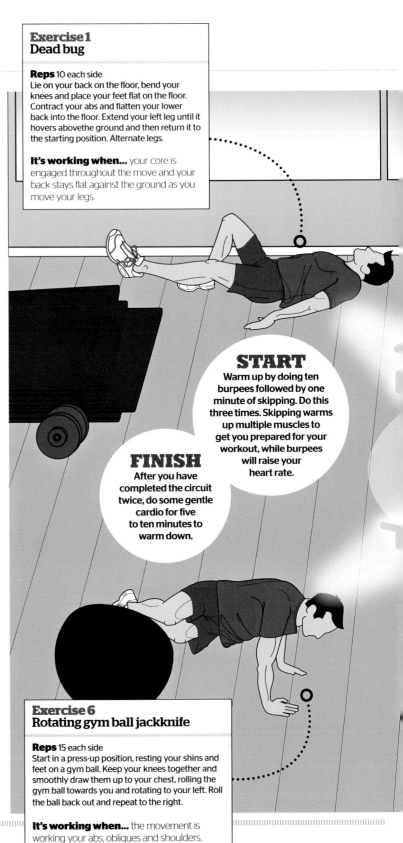

Exercise 1
Dead bug

Reps 10 each side
Lie on your back on the floor, bend your knees and place your feet flat on the floor. Contract your abs and flatten your lower back into the floor. Extend your left leg until it hovers abovethe ground and then return it to the starting position. Alternate legs.

It's working when... your core is engaged throughout the move and your back stays flat against the ground as you move your legs.

START
Warm up by doing ten burpees followed by one minute of skipping. Do this three times. Skipping warms up multiple muscles to get you prepared for your workout, while burpees will raise your heart rate.

FINISH
After you have completed the circuit twice, do some gentle cardio for five to ten minutes to warm down.

Exercise 6
Rotating gym ball jackknife

Reps 15 each side
Start in a press-up position, resting your shins and feet on a gym ball. Keep your knees together and smoothly draw them up to your chest, rolling the gym ball towards you and rotating to your left. Roll the ball back out and repeat to the right.

It's working when... the movement is working your abs, obliques and shoulders.

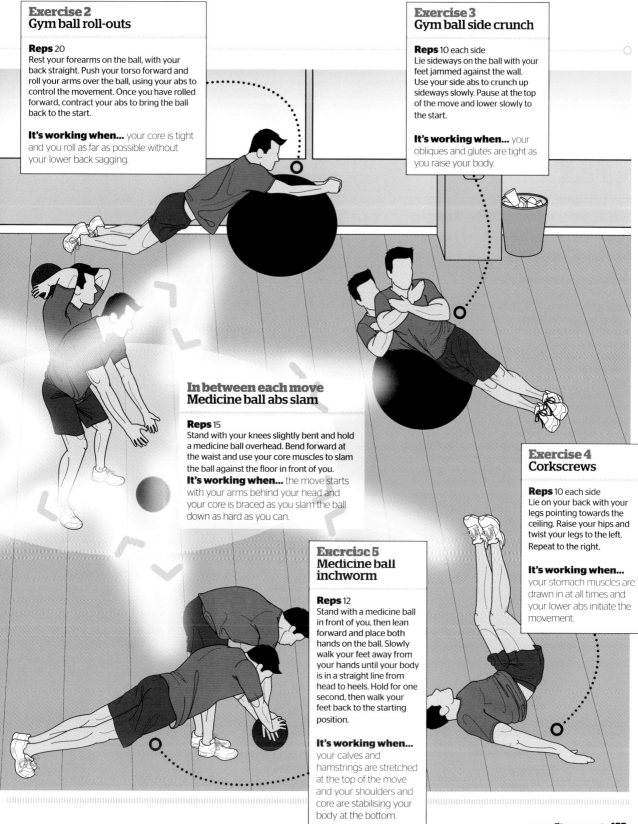

Exercise 2
Gym ball roll-outs

Reps 20
Rest your forearms on the ball, with your back straight. Push your torso forward and roll your arms over the ball, using your abs to control the movement. Once you have rolled forward, contract your abs to bring the ball back to the start.

It's working when... your core is tight and you roll as far as possible without your lower back sagging.

Exercise 3
Gym ball side crunch

Reps 10 each side
Lie sideways on the ball with your feet jammed against the wall. Use your side abs to crunch up sideways slowly. Pause at the top of the move and lower slowly to the start.

It's working when... your obliques and glutes are tight as you raise your body.

In between each move
Medicine ball abs slam

Reps 15
Stand with your knees slightly bent and hold a medicine ball overhead. Bend forward at the waist and use your core muscles to slam the ball against the floor in front of you.
It's working when... the move starts with your arms behind your head and your core is braced as you slam the ball down as hard as you can.

Exercise 4
Corkscrews

Reps 10 each side
Lie on your back with your legs pointing towards the ceiling. Raise your hips and twist your legs to the left. Repeat to the right.

It's working when... your stomach muscles are drawn in at all times and your lower abs initiate the movement.

Exercise 5
Medicine ball inchworm

Reps 12
Stand with a medicine ball in front of you, then lean forward and place both hands on the ball. Slowly walk your feet away from your hands until your body is in a straight line from head to heels. Hold for one second, then walk your feet back to the starting position.

It's working when... your calves and hamstrings are stretched at the top of the move and your shoulders and core are stabilising your body at the bottom.

Fat Loss ▶
Speed Circuit

Game on

Kick your body into shape with this calorie-burning football circuit

How it works

Although football is a great sport, taking a keen interest in the game can mean that you spend an unhealthy amount of time in the pub or stuck to the sofa.

To stop the booze and junk food taking its toll on your gut, try this heart-racing circuit that allows you to blitz calories and protect against injury in less than half an hour.

You'll find that the sprints get your heart rate up quicker than charging across the pub as the ball hits the net, while the plyometric exercises help

you produce more power when you are actually on the pitch. There are also moves to help you strengthen your ankles and core, and improve your balance, which will make you less susceptible to injury.

Do all the exercises in order with as little rest as you can between each move. Once you have completed one circuit, rest for two minutes before repeating it. You then have permission to join your fellow supporters for a well deserved pint.

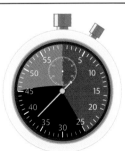

Time per session
25 minutes
Calorie burn
450

Exercise 1
Burpee into fast feet

Time 60 seconds
Get into a press-up position with your hands on the football. Bring your knees towards your chest and then jump up off the ground, lifting the ball above your head. As you land, run on the spot as fast as you can, counting for ten before performing another burpee.

It's working when... the movement of your feet is a blur and your heart rate is through the roof.

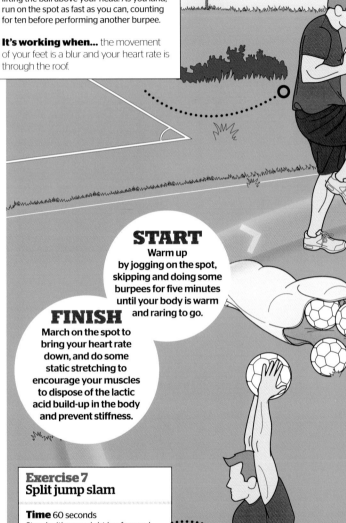

START
Warm up by jogging on the spot, skipping and doing some burpees for five minutes until your body is warm and raring to go.

FINISH
March on the spot to bring your heart rate down, and do some static stretching to encourage your muscles to dispose of the lactic acid build-up in the body and prevent stiffness.

Exercise 7
Split jump slam

Time 60 seconds
Stand with your right leg forward and your left leg behind you in a split squat position. Hold the ball above your head. Bend into a lunge, rotate your torso to the right and slam the ball on the ground outside of your right knee. Jump up, switch legs in mid-air, catch the ball and bring it back above your head.

It's working when... your quads are burning while your shoulders, core, glutes and calves co-ordinate the move.

Illustrations **Stuart Holmes@Illustrationweb** The amount of calories burned will vary depending on your bodyweight and ×tness level

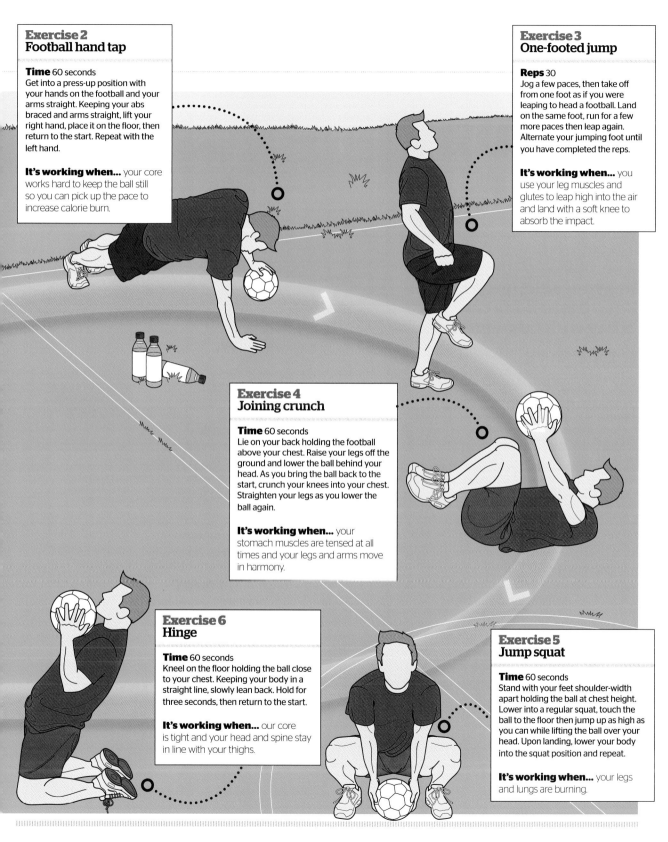

Exercise 2
Football hand tap

Time 60 seconds
Get into a press-up position with your hands on the football and your arms straight. Keeping your abs braced and arms straight, lift your right hand, place it on the floor, then return to the start. Repeat with the left hand.

It's working when... your core works hard to keep the ball still so you can pick up the pace to increase calorie burn.

Exercise 3
One-footed jump

Reps 30
Jog a few paces, then take off from one foot as if you were leaping to head a football. Land on the same foot, run for a few more paces then leap again. Alternate your jumping foot until you have completed the reps.

It's working when... you use your leg muscles and glutes to leap high into the air and land with a soft knee to absorb the impact.

Exercise 4
Joining crunch

Time 60 seconds
Lie on your back holding the football above your chest. Raise your legs off the ground and lower the ball behind your head. As you bring the ball back to the start, crunch your knees into your chest. Straighten your legs as you lower the ball again.

It's working when... your stomach muscles are tensed at all times and your legs and arms move in harmony.

Exercise 6
Hinge

Time 60 seconds
Kneel on the floor holding the ball close to your chest. Keeping your body in a straight line, slowly lean back. Hold for three seconds, then return to the start.

It's working when... our core is tight and your head and spine stay in line with your thighs.

Exercise 5
Jump squat

Time 60 seconds
Stand with your feet shoulder-width apart holding the ball at chest height. Lower into a regular squat, touch the ball to the floor then jump up as high as you can while lifting the ball over your head. Upon landing, lower your body into the squat position and repeat.

It's working when... your legs and lungs are burning.

Burning in the sun

Not your skin, but your fat. Keep the holiday calories at bay with this workout

How it works

Being on holiday usually means developing an unhealthy relationship with the sun lounger and the cocktail menu. So see off the guilt and the flab that come with gorging on local delicacies and sitting on the beach nine hours a day with MF's quickfire beach-based, fat-burning circuit.

Most of the moves in this routine are based on plyometric exercises, which burn calories and build lean muscle fast. Working out on sand provides less stability, making the simplest of moves much tougher. Running on sand can also burn over 50 per cent more calories than running on a flat surface would, meaning you don't have to waste precious holiday time with long workouts or punish yourself with an epic workout schedule when your break is over.

Perform the exercises in order, with a 40-second run between moves.

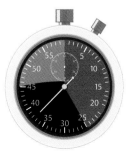

Time per session

30 minutes

Calorie burn

400

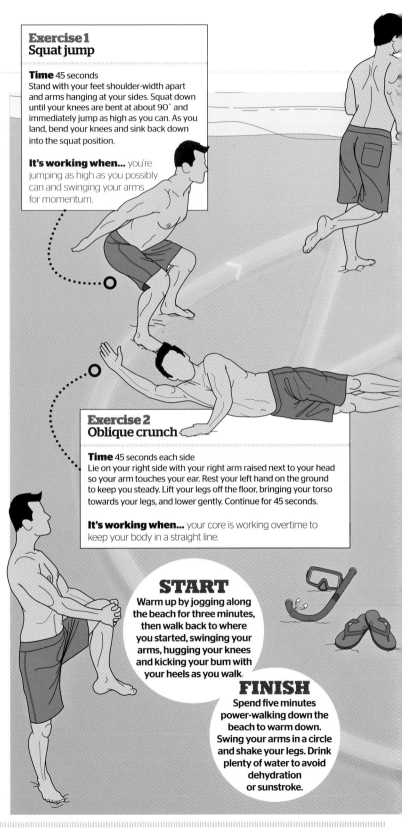

Exercise 1
Squat jump

Time 45 seconds
Stand with your feet shoulder-width apart and arms hanging at your sides. Squat down until your knees are bent at about 90˚ and immediately jump as high as you can. As you land, bend your knees and sink back down into the squat position.

It's working when... you're jumping as high as you possibly can and swinging your arms for momentum.

Exercise 2
Oblique crunch

Time 45 seconds each side
Lie on your right side with your right arm raised next to your head so your arm touches your ear. Rest your left hand on the ground to keep you steady. Lift your legs off the floor, bringing your torso towards your legs, and lower gently. Continue for 45 seconds.

It's working when... your core is working overtime to keep your body in a straight line.

START
Warm up by jogging along the beach for three minutes, then walk back to where you started, swinging your arms, hugging your knees and kicking your bum with your heels as you walk.

FINISH
Spend five minutes power-walking down the beach to warm down. Swing your arms in a circle and shake your legs. Drink plenty of water to avoid dehydration or sunstroke.

Illustrations **Stuart Holmes@illustrationweb** The number of calories burned will vary depending on your bodyweight and ×thess level

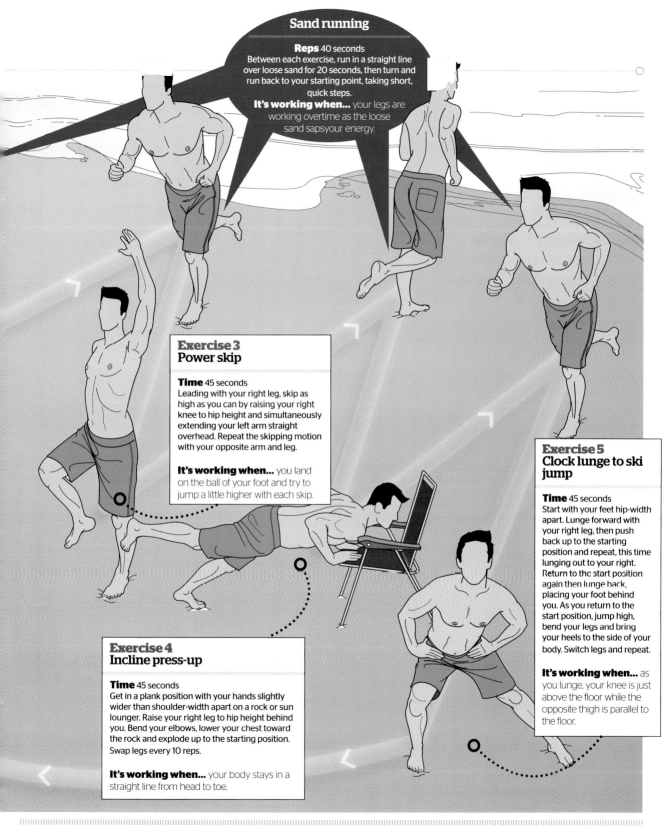

Sand running

Reps 40 seconds
Between each exercise, run in a straight line over loose sand for 20 seconds, then turn and run back to your starting point, taking short, quick steps.
It's working when... your legs are working overtime as the loose sand saps your energy.

Exercise 3
Power skip

Time 45 seconds
Leading with your right leg, skip as high as you can by raising your right knee to hip height and simultaneously extending your left arm straight overhead. Repeat the skipping motion with your opposite arm and leg.

It's working when... you land on the ball of your foot and try to jump a little higher with each skip.

Exercise 5
Clock lunge to ski jump

Time 45 seconds
Start with your feet hip-width apart. Lunge forward with your right leg, then push back up to the starting position and repeat, this time lunging out to your right. Return to the start position again then lunge back, placing your foot behind you. As you return to the start position, jump high, bend your legs and bring your heels to the side of your body. Switch legs and repeat.

It's working when... as you lunge, your knee is just above the floor while the opposite thigh is parallel to the floor.

Exercise 4
Incline press-up

Time 45 seconds
Get in a plank position with your hands slightly wider than shoulder-width apart on a rock or sun lounger. Raise your right leg to hip height behind you. Bend your elbows, lower your chest toward the rock and explode up to the starting position. Swap legs every 10 reps.

It's working when... your body stays in a straight line from head to toe.

Hit the trail

Get outside and lose weight with this 30-minute fat-frying park circuit

How it works

When the sun is shining there is no reason to be sweating it out in the gym – instead it's time to take your workouts al fresco. But just doing a few laps of your local park simply won't cut it. You need to string together bodyweight exercises such as burpees, press-ups and lunges into a circuit which will not only push your heart rate and metabolism through the roof but to also add some variety, agility and fun to your workout.

A park workout is also good news for your muscles. By working against the natural elements of the great outdoors you will switch on new muscles, as they respond to a new environment while burning more calories. Research shows exercising outdoors can boost your core stability, cut tension and improve mental health.

Do all the exercises in order with as little rest as you can between each move. Run between stations and try and perform as many reps as you possibly can in the time limit.

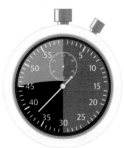

Time per session
30 minutes
Calorie burn
450

*Illustrations **Sudden Impact** The amount of calories burned will vary depending on your bodyweight and ×tness level*

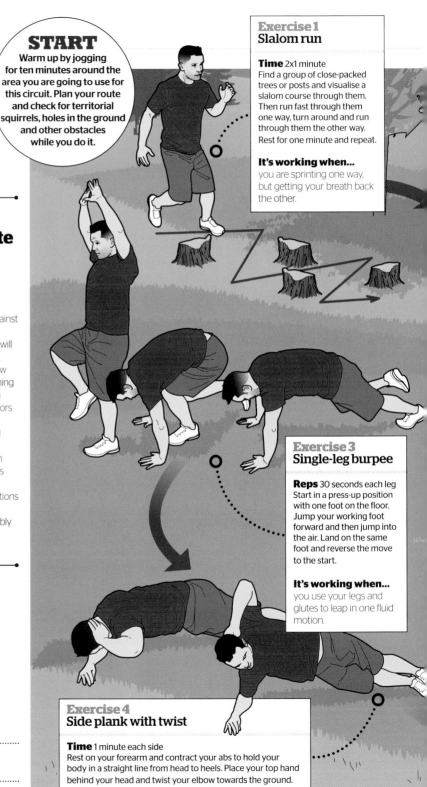

START
Warm up by jogging for ten minutes around the area you are going to use for this circuit. Plan your route and check for territorial squirrels, holes in the ground and other obstacles while you do it.

Exercise 1
Slalom run

Time 2x1 minute
Find a group of close-packed trees or posts and visualise a slalom course through them. Then run fast through them one way, turn around and run through them the other way. Rest for one minute and repeat.

It's working when...
you are sprinting one way, but getting your breath back the other.

Exercise 3
Single-leg burpee

Reps 30 seconds each leg
Start in a press-up position with one foot on the floor. Jump your working foot forward and then jump into the air. Land on the same foot and reverse the move to the start.

It's working when...
you use your legs and glutes to leap in one fluid motion.

Exercise 4
Side plank with twist

Time 1 minute each side
Rest on your forearm and contract your abs to hold your body in a straight line from head to heels. Place your top hand behind your head and twist your elbow towards the ground.

It's working when... your abs are tight and your hips are high throughout the whole move.

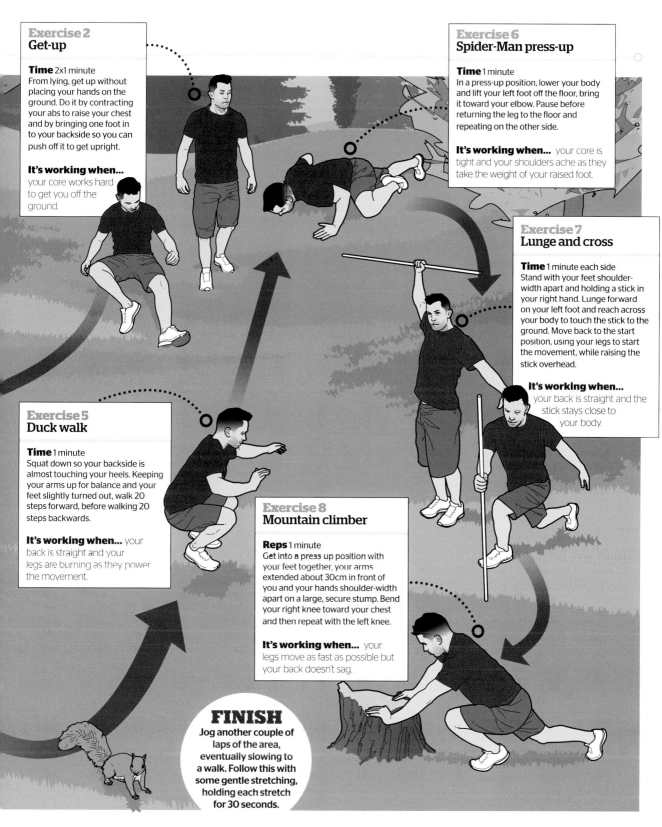

Exercise 2
Get-up

Time 2x1 minute
From lying, get up without placing your hands on the ground. Do it by contracting your abs to raise your chest and by bringing one foot in to your backside so you can push off it to get upright.

It's working when... your core works hard to get you off the ground.

Exercise 6
Spider-Man press-up

Time 1 minute
In a press-up position, lower your body and lift your left foot off the floor, bring it toward your elbow. Pause before returning the leg to the floor and repeating on the other side.

It's working when... your core is tight and your shoulders ache as they take the weight of your raised foot.

Exercise 7
Lunge and cross

Time 1 minute each side
Stand with your feet shoulder-width apart and holding a stick in your right hand. Lunge forward on your left foot and reach across your body to touch the stick to the ground. Move back to the start position, using your legs to start the movement, while raising the stick overhead.

It's working when... your back is straight and the stick stays close to your body.

Exercise 5
Duck walk

Time 1 minute
Squat down so your backside is almost touching your heels. Keeping your arms up for balance and your feet slightly turned out, walk 20 steps forward, before walking 20 steps backwards.

It's working when... your back is straight and your legs are burning as they power the movement.

Exercise 8
Mountain climber

Reps 1 minute
Get into a press up position with your feet together, your arms extended about 30cm in front of you and your hands shoulder-width apart on a large, secure stump. Bend your right knee toward your chest and then repeat with the left knee.

It's working when... your legs move as fast as possible but your back doesn't sag.

FINISH
Jog another couple of laps of the area, eventually slowing to a walk. Follow this with some gentle stretching, holding each stretch for 30 seconds.

Rise & shine

Can't find the time to exercise? Get up earlier and do it before your busy life takes over

How it works

After a long day at work, it's all too tempting to forgo the gym and slump in front of Sky Sports. You'll feel a lot better about doing this if you've already done a vigorous workout. Just set your alarm 30 minutes earlier and take the chance to burn hundreds of calories with a high-intensity circuit first thing in the morning before the chaos of your day gets going.

Your testosterone levels are at the their highest point in the morning, which makes it easier to build muscle and burn fat. Since you won't have eaten much you'll also blast loads of fat.

Do all the exercises in order with just ten seconds' rest between each move. Once you have completed one circuit, rest for two minutes before repeating it another three times. You should then treat yourself to a cool shower to increase the blood flow to the muscles and stave off muscle soreness. You may yelp with shock but your muscles will thank you for it.

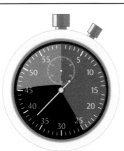

Time per session
25 minutes
Calorie burn
400

Illustrations **Sudden Impact** The amount of calories burned will vary depending on your bodyweight and ×tness level

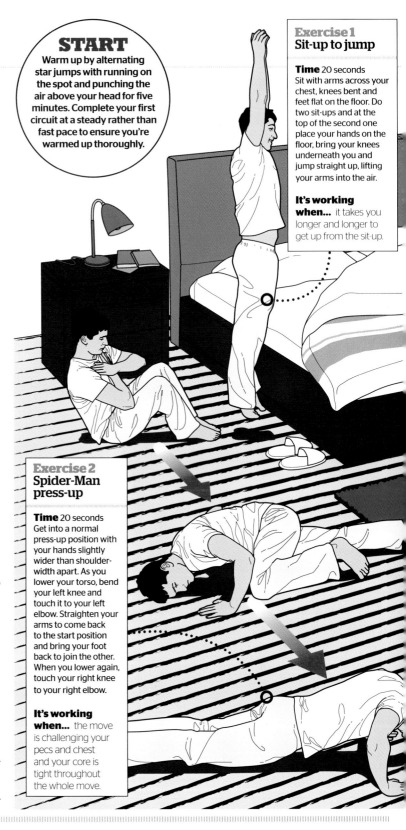

START
Warm up by alternating star jumps with running on the spot and punching the air above your head for five minutes. Complete your first circuit at a steady rather than fast pace to ensure you're warmed up thoroughly.

Exercise 1
Sit-up to jump

Time 20 seconds
Sit with arms across your chest, knees bent and feet flat on the floor. Do two sit-ups and at the top of the second one place your hands on the floor, bring your knees underneath you and jump straight up, lifting your arms into the air.

It's working when... it takes you longer and longer to get up from the sit-up.

Exercise 2
Spider-Man press-up

Time 20 seconds
Get into a normal press-up position with your hands slightly wider than shoulder-width apart. As you lower your torso, bend your left knee and touch it to your left elbow. Straighten your arms to come back to the start position and bring your foot back to join the other. When you lower again, touch your right knee to your right elbow.

It's working when... the move is challenging your pecs and chest and your core is tight throughout the whole move.

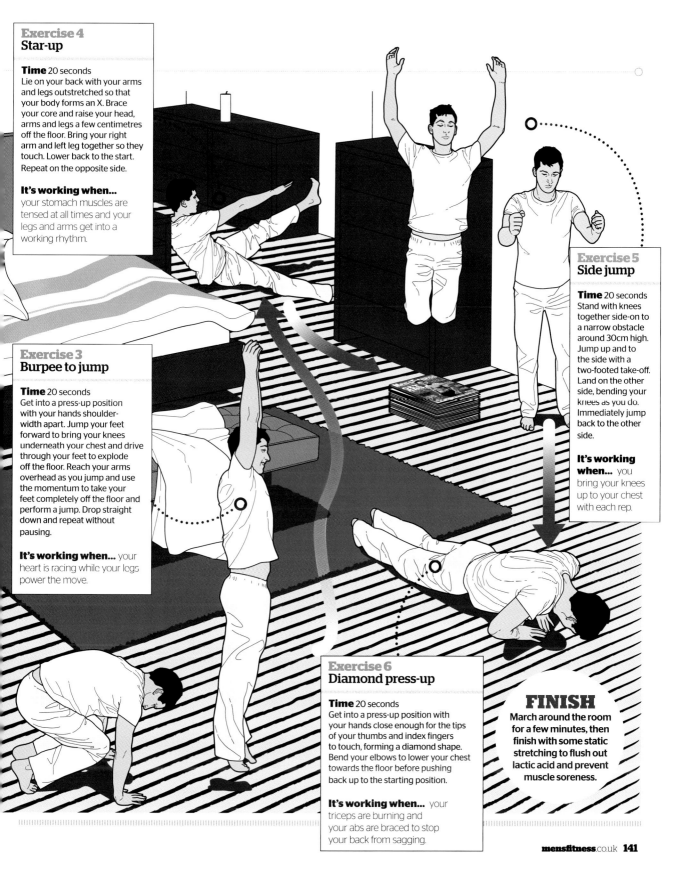

Exercise 4
Star-up

Time 20 seconds
Lie on your back with your arms and legs outstretched so that your body forms an X. Brace your core and raise your head, arms and legs a few centimetres off the floor. Bring your right arm and left leg together so they touch. Lower back to the start. Repeat on the opposite side.

It's working when...
your stomach muscles are tensed at all times and your legs and arms get into a working rhythm.

Exercise 3
Burpee to jump

Time 20 seconds
Get into a press-up position with your hands shoulder-width apart. Jump your feet forward to bring your knees underneath your chest and drive through your feet to explode off the floor. Reach your arms overhead as you jump and use the momentum to take your feet completely off the floor and perform a jump. Drop straight down and repeat without pausing.

It's working when... your heart is racing while your legs power the move.

Exercise 5
Side jump

Time 20 seconds
Stand with knees together side-on to a narrow obstacle around 30cm high. Jump up and to the side with a two-footed take-off. Land on the other side, bending your knees as you do. Immediately jump back to the other side.

It's working when... you bring your knees up to your chest with each rep.

Exercise 6
Diamond press-up

Time 20 seconds
Get into a press-up position with your hands close enough for the tips of your thumbs and index fingers to touch, forming a diamond shape. Bend your elbows to lower your chest towards the floor before pushing back up to the starting position.

It's working when... your triceps are burning and your abs are braced to stop your back from sagging.

FINISH
March around the room for a few minutes, then finish with some static stretching to flush out lactic acid and prevent muscle soreness.

Fat Loss ▶
Speed Circuit

Home gains

This intense circuit will deliver explosive strength fast and burn fat – all in the comfort of your own home

How it works

There are plenty of advantages to working out at home rather than at the gym. You can do it whenever you've got the time, you can blast out your own music and there are no sweaty blokes with personal hygiene issues.

You might not have a full set of free weights and machines, but this shouldn't stop you. There's a vast array of bodyweight exercises – such as the ones selected for this circuit – that will keep your workouts interesting. Meanwhile, the pyramid reps will keep your heart rate high and help build muscle endurance, giving this circuit all the ingredients required to burn fat and build muscle.

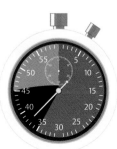

Time per session

35 minutes

Calorie burn

400

*Illustrations **Stuart Holmes@Illustrationweb** The amount of calories burned will vary depending on your bodyweight and ×tness level*

PYRAMID REPS
After warming up, do Exercise 1. Rest for 30 seconds and then repeat Exercise 1, then without resting do Exercise 2. Rest for 30 seconds before doing Exercises 1, 2 and 3 without rest, then rest for 30 seconds. Continue the sequence, adding an exercise each time.

Exercise 1
Shadowboxing

Time 1 minute
Get into a boxing stance and start to throw punches at an imaginary opponent. Alternate hands, and combine jabs with uppercuts and hooks.

It's working when... you are moving around and practising your footwork as you throw strong punches.

START
Warm-up by jogging on the spot for one minute before running up and down the stairs five times. Then spend five minutes doing dynamic squats and lunges.

FINISH
Spend at least five minutes cooling down. Stretch to help reduce muscle injury, stiffness and soreness.

Exercise 6
Standing calf raises

Time 1 minute
Place the balls of your feet on the edge of a step with your feet shoulder-width apart. Lower your heels as far as you can, then rise back up onto your toes.

It's working when... your core is working hard to keep your balance and your calves are burning.

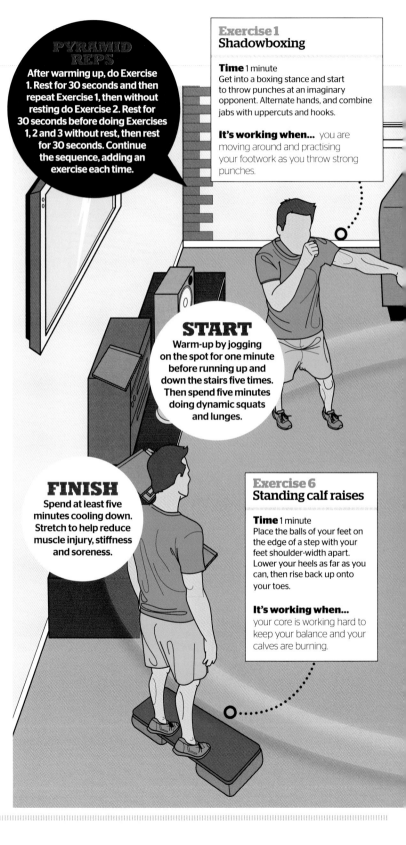

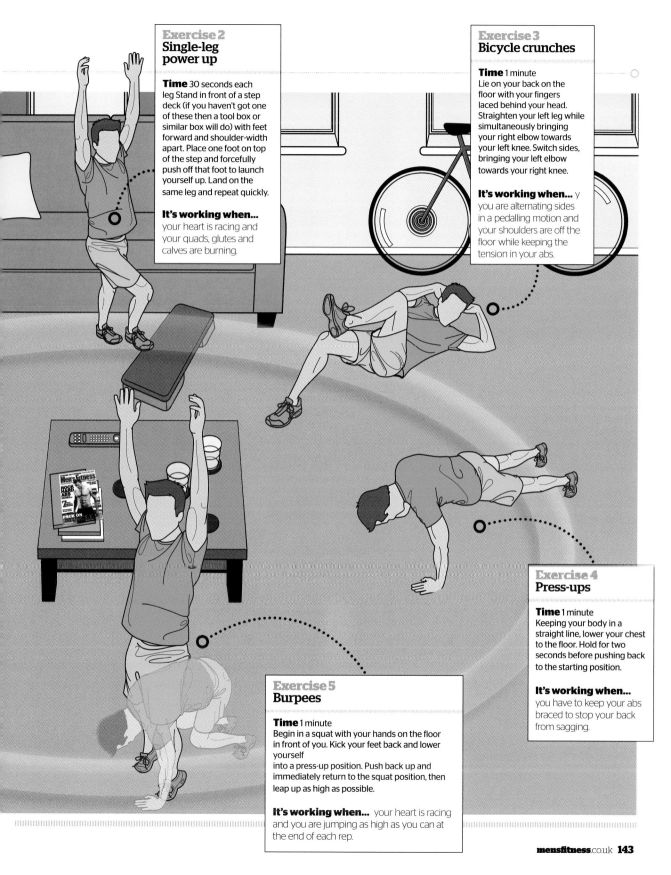

Exercise 2
Single-leg power up

Time 30 seconds each leg Stand in front of a step deck (if you haven't got one of these then a tool box or similar box will do) with feet forward and shoulder-width apart. Place one foot on top of the step and forcefully push off that foot to launch yourself up. Land on the same leg and repeat quickly.

It's working when... your heart is racing and your quads, glutes and calves are burning.

Exercise 3
Bicycle crunches

Time 1 minute Lie on your back on the floor with your fingers laced behind your head. Straighten your left leg while simultaneously bringing your right elbow towards your left knee. Switch sides, bringing your left elbow towards your right knee.

It's working when... y you are alternating sides in a pedalling motion and your shoulders are off the floor while keeping the tension in your abs.

Exercise 4
Press-ups

Time 1 minute Keeping your body in a straight line, lower your chest to the floor. Hold for two seconds before pushing back to the starting position.

It's working when... you have to keep your abs braced to stop your back from sagging.

Exercise 5
Burpees

Time 1 minute Begin in a squat with your hands on the floor in front of you. Kick your feet back and lower yourself into a press-up position. Push back up and immediately return to the squat position, then leap up as high as possible.

It's working when... your heart is racing and you are jumping as high as you can at the end of each rep.

Speed Circuit

Travel training

Your exercise regime doesn't have to take a break when you're away from home. Stay lean with this do-it-anywhere circuit

How it works

Not every hotel has a state-of-the-art gym, but that doesn't mean you should develop an unhealthy relationship with the mini-bar instead. This workout allows you to work on your fitness and burn fat without packing your dumb-bells and gym ball. Working on an unstable platform such as a bed

or pillow, according to US research, will make your leg and hip muscles work up to 13 per cent harder as they strive to keep your balance. If you do crash to the floor and disturb other residents, MF takes no responsibility for the arguments – just don't do it in the middle of the night...

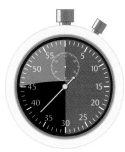

Time per session
30 minutes

Calorie burn
450

Illustrations **Stuart Holmes@illustrationweb** The amount of calories burned will vary depending on your bodyweight and ×tness level

Exercise 1
Pillow sprint

Time 4x30 seconds
Place a pillow on the floor and stand on it. Sprint on the spot as fast as you can, driving your legs and pumping your arms. Rest for ten seconds between each 30-second sprint.

It's working when... the muscles in your lower body are working flat out and the pillow is sapping your energy.

START
Get your blood circulating by doing five minutes of jogging on the spot, jumping jacks and heel flicks. Then do some squats, walking lunges and press-ups back to back for five minutes to improve your co-ordination and the elasticity of your muscles.

FINISH
Once you have completed one circuit, rest for two minutes before repeating it.

Exercise 7
Reverse chair crunch

Reps 20 each side
Sit on a chair (not leaning against the back) with your shoulders back. Push your legs out, keeping them under control, then pull your knees in to one side of your chest. Push them out again and pull them in to the other side.

It's working when... your lower abs and hip flexors are working together to crunch your knees into your chest.

Exercise 6
Superman

Reps 20
Lie on your front with your arms out in front of you. Raise your arms, chest and feet off the floor. Hold this position for three seconds, then lower back slowly.

It's working when... your lower back is doing most of the work and your glutes are squeezed tight at the top of the move.

Exercise 2
Single-leg squat

Reps 15 each leg
Stand on a pillow on one leg with the other leg held out behind you. Bend your knee to lower your body, keeping your back straight and your knee in line with your foot. Squat down as low as possible and then drive up through your heel back to the starting position.

It's working when... your hips and leg muscles are working overtime to keep you balanced.

Exercise 3
Step-up

Reps 25 each side
Stand in front of the bed and step up onto it with your right foot, driving up and placing your left foot beside it. Step back down with the trailing leg and repeat as before on the other leg. Continue to alternate legs.

It's working when... your movement is fast and your quads and glutes are burning as they power the move.

Exercise 5
Side plank

Reps 30 seconds each side
Lie on your left side, resting your weight on your left forearm and placing your right hand on your uppermost thigh. With your right foot resting on top of your left, contract your abs and raise your hips so that your body forms a straight line from your ankles to your neck. Hold for 30 seconds, then swap sides.

It's working when... your obliques are taut and your core and shoulders are working overtime to maintain balance.

Exercise 4
Feet-up triceps dip

Reps 20
Sit on the edge of the bed with your feet on a chair. Place the heels of your hands on the bed and slide your backside off the edge. Bend your elbows back, and slowly lower your body toward the floor. Keep your elbows tucked in. Push back up until your arms are straight.

It's working when... your core muscles are working hard to maintain perfect form throughout.

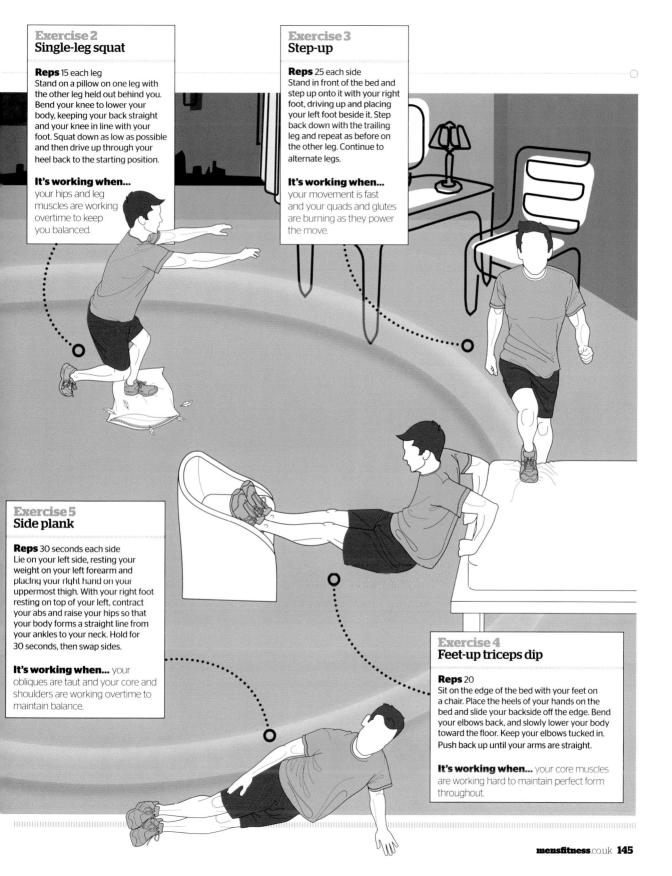

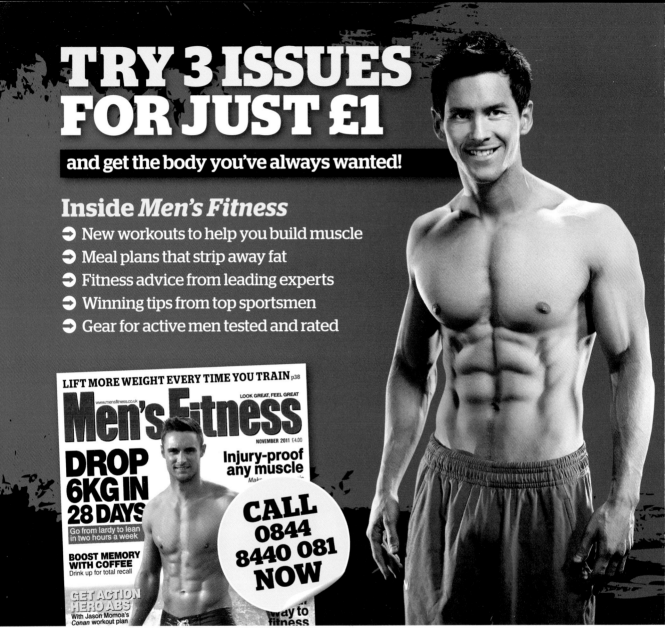